OF01032

Revision Questions for Paediatrics

EMQs with answers explained

OLAMIDE OREKUNRIN MBBS
Research Fellow
Jikei Hospital, Tokyo

and

HELEN CHAPLIN MBChB, MRCPCH
Paediatric Speciality Registrar
New Cross Hospital, Wolverhampton

Radcliffe Publishing
Oxford • New York

Radcliffe Publishing Ltd
18 Marcham Road
Abingdon
Oxon OX14 1AA
United Kingdom

www.radcliffe-oxford.com
Electronic catalogue and worldwide online ordering facility.

British Library Cataloguing in Publication Data
A catalogue record for this book is available from the British Library.

ISBN-13: 978 184619 376 7

The information contained within this book was obtained by the authors from
reliable sources. However, while every effort has been made to ensure its accuracy,
no responsibility for loss, damage or injury occasioned to any person acting or
refraining from action as a result of information contained herein can be accepted
by the publisher or the authors.

The paper used for the text pages of this book
is FSC certified. FSC (The Forest Stewardship
Council) is an international network to promote
responsible management of the world's forests.

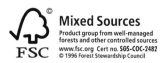

Mixed Sources
Product group from well-managed
forests and other controlled sources
www.fsc.org Cert no. SGS-COC-2482
© 1996 Forest Stewardship Council

Typeset by Pindar NZ, Auckland, New Zealand
Printed and bound by TJI Digital, Padstow, Cornwall, UK

Contents

Preface   vi
About the authors   vii
List of contributors   viii

Chapter 1
Neonatology   1

Chapter 2
Neurology and development   13

Chapter 3
Immunology and infectious disease   23

Chapter 4
Gastroenterology and endocrinology   37

Chapter 5
Cardiology and respiratory disease   51

Chapter 6
Orthopaedics and rheumatology   63

Chapter 7
Haematology and oncology   73

Chapter 8
Nephrology and urology   85

Chapter 9
Emergency paediatrics and non-accidental injury   99

Chapter 10
Public health and statistics   115

Index   127

Preface

This book is intended primarily for medical students who are preparing for their exams in paediatrics. It is intended as a revision tool, and includes many topics that are frequently asked in paediatric exams. It gives detailed answers to enable the student to learn through practising the questions.

Different people like to adopt different revision plans. We advise that students try a chapter at a time, attempting the questions and then marking them and reading the answers at the back of the book. They should then spend some time reading around each subject, before trying the questions again. And then note the improvement!

The questions are set in an extended matching question (EMQ) format. A number of medical schools are now examining students using EMQs, so practising this style of question is helpful. In addition, EMQs feature prominently in postgraduate examinations, so would also be useful to those preparing for postgraduate examinations such as the Diploma in Child Health (DCH) and Membership of the Royal College of Paediatrics and Child Health (MRCPCH).

And finally ... good luck in the exam!

Olamide Orekunrin
Helen Chaplin
June 2010

About the authors

Dr Ola Orekunrin MBBS
Ola qualified in 2008 from the Hull York Medical School, having maintained a special interest in paediatrics throughout her studies. After completing her foundation training, she was awarded the prestigious Japanese MEXT Fellowship in 2010, and is currently completing her research thesis, on the role of iPS cell-based therapies for children with genetic diseases, at Jikei University, Tokyo. She has recently combined her love of rotary-wing flying with her passion for improving the outcomes of paediatric trauma in Africa by starting up West Africa's first air ambulance service.

Dr Helen Chaplin MBChB, MRCPCH
Helen Chaplin qualified in 2003 from the University of Birmingham, and has worked within paediatrics since 2004. She has trained in the Midlands area of the UK, in Birmingham, Derby, Coventry and Wolverhampton. She became a Member of the Royal College of Paediatrics and Child Health in 2007, and is currently working as a Paediatric Specialty Registrar in Wolverhampton and is specialising in community paediatrics. Coming from a family of teachers, Helen has a particular interest in education, and regularly enjoys leading a variety of paediatric teaching sessions.

List of contributors

Dr Guy Millman MBBS, MRCPCH
Consultant Paediatrician
York District Hospital
Neonatology
Neurology and development

Dr Vinod Patel MBBS, MD
Consultant Physician and Associate Professor in Endocrinology and
Diabetes
George Eliot Hospital
Nuneaton
Emergency paediatrics and non-accidental injury

Dr Sarah Thompson MBChB, MRCPCH
Consultant Paediatrician
University Hospital North Staffordshire
Haematology and oncology

Miss Lucy Cooper MBBS, MRCS
Specialist Registrar, Trauma and Orthopaedics
Alder Hey Children's Hospital
Liverpool
Emergency paediatrics and non-accidental injury
Orthopaedics and rheumatology

Dr Damiete Harry MBBS, BSc
Senior House Officer, Surgery
Barts and the London NHS Trust
Emergency paediatrics and non-accidental injury

Dr Jessie Morgan MBBS
Senior House Officer, General Medicine
Hull and East Yorkshire Hospitals NHS Trust
Public health and statistics

Dr Lucy Rapp MBBS
Foundation Year Two Doctor
University Hospitals Coventry and Warwickshire
Cardiology and respiratory disease

Dr Andrea Warnock MBBS
Foundation Year Two Doctor
University Hospital of North Staffordshire
Haematology and oncology

This book is dedicated to my sister, Busola,
who I know would have been so proud to see my name in print.
Ola Orekunrin

I dedicate this book to my dad, Martin Chaplin,
from whom I inherited my love of teaching.
Helen Chaplin

1 Neonatology

QUESTIONS

1) From the list of options below, please select the most likely diagnosis for each of the following scenarios concerning newborns. Each option may be used more than once.

   A. Down's syndrome
   B. Transient tachypnoea of the newborn
   C. Respiratory distress syndrome
   D. Hypoglycaemia
   E. Transposition of the great arteries
   F. Neonatal lupus erythematosus
   G. Neonatal abstinence syndrome
   H. Intrauterine growth deficiency
   I. Bronchopneumonia
   J. Tetralogy of Fallot
   K. Monosomy
   L. Trisomy 18

   1. A full-term baby boy is born by elective Caesarean section. He develops signs of respiratory distress at 30 minutes of age.

   2. A full-term baby girl develops central cyanosis a few hours after birth. She was treated with prostaglandin therapy.

   3. A term newborn develops hyperirritability, gastrointestinal dysfunction, sneezing and exaggerated reflexes at 72 hours of age.

4. A baby boy was stillborn at 37 weeks' gestation. He had rocker-bottom foot and overlapping fingers.

5. A newborn has a persistent bradycardia. An ECG confirms a complete heart block.

2) From the list of options below, please select the most appropriate diagnosis for each of the following scenarios and statements concerning premature neonates. Each option may be used more than once.

A. Patent ductus arteriosus
B. Periventricular leukomalacia
C. Hirschsprung's disease
D. Chronic lung disease
E. Intraventricular haemorrhage
F. Monosomy
G. Respiratory distress syndrome
H. Retinopathy of prematurity
I. Necrotising enterocolitis
J. Haemoglobinopathy
K. Apnoea of prematurity
L. Bronchopneumonia

1. A 3-day-old baby who was born at 30 weeks' gestation shows no signs of respiratory distress, but has recurrent pauses in his breathing that last for more than 20 seconds.

2. A 2-week-old baby girl who was born prematurely at 28 weeks' gestation becomes increasingly lethargic, with marked feed intolerance. On examination, her abdomen is swollen and tender.

3. This condition may be caused by the acute or chronic effects of oxygen toxicity on the blood vessels.

4. Oliguria is a recognised side-effect of the treatment for this condition.

5. A baby boy is born at 26 weeks' gestation. When he is 10 weeks old he still requires nasal prong oxygen. His X-rays show a sponge-like appearance, with areas of lung opacification.

3) From the list of options below, please select the most likely diagnosis for each of the following scenarios concerning jaundice in the neonatal period. Each option may be used more than once.

A. Gallstones
B. Physiological jaundice
C. Rhesus incompatibility
D. Thalassaemia
E. Kernicterus
F. G6PD deficiency
G. Hydrops fetalis
H. Intraventricular haemorrhage
I. Breast milk jaundice
J. ABO incompatibility
K. Pyruvate kinase deficiency
L. Liver failure

1. A baby girl is born at 35 weeks' gestation by Caesarean section. She develops jaundice on day 2 with a maximum bilirubin level of 200 mmol/l on day 3. The jaundice resolves by day 7.

2. A baby boy is born by emergency Caesarean section at 37 weeks' gestation due to rising maternal anti-D titres and pleural effusions seen on the baby's antenatal scan. He is very oedematous at delivery, and the cord bilirubin level is 50 mmol/l.

3. A baby boy is born at term by normal vaginal delivery. His mother's blood group is O Rhesus positive. He is observed to be jaundiced at 18 hours of age.

4. A baby boy of Mediterranean origin is born at term by normal vaginal delivery after an uncomplicated pregnancy. He is discharged home the following day after a normal baby check. He presents again at 14 days of age with severe haemolytic jaundice.

5. A baby boy is born at term by normal vaginal delivery. The pregnancy was not booked, as the mother denied knowing that she was pregnant. The baby was found to be significantly jaundiced at 12 hours of age, and his bilirubin level increased to 550 mmol/l, despite phototherapy. He developed irritability, hypertonia and back arching.

4) From the list of options below, please select the most likely diagnosis for each of the following scenarios, which describe possible findings at the newborn baby check. Each option may be used more than once.

A. Prader–Willi syndrome
B. Edwards' syndrome
C. Erb's palsy
D. Congenital cataract
E. Absent anus
F. Turner's syndrome
G. Klumpke's palsy
H. Viral gastroenteritis
I. Cleft palate
J. Spina bifida
K. Cystic fibrosis
L. Congenital hypothyroidism

1. A baby boy was born at term by normal vaginal delivery, and had a birth weight of 4.9 kg. Neonatal examination revealed an abnormal Moro reflex. The Moro reflex was normal on the left side, but there was very little movement of the right arm. There was positive hand grasp bilaterally.

2. A baby girl who was born at term is found to have puffy feet and a cystic hygroma at her neonatal examination.

3. A 1-day-old term baby boy has not been feeding well, despite looking hungry. He also vomited from his nostrils.

4. A baby boy born at term has not passed meconium by 36 hours of age. There is no visible anorectal malformation on direct inspection, he has vomited several times, and his abdomen appears distended.

5. A baby girl is born at term by normal vaginal delivery. On direct ophthalmoscopy, no red reflex is seen in either eye.

ANSWERS

1) B, E, G, L, F

1. B. Transient tachypnoea of the newborn

Transient tachypnoea of the newborn (TTN) is usually a self-limiting condition that is characterised by tachypnoea, mild recession, grunting and occasionally hypoxia. It is usually noted in larger premature infants or term infants who have been delivered by Caesarean section or precipitous delivery. Infants born to diabetic mothers and those with poor respiratory drive due to placental passage of analgesic drugs are also at risk. Chest radiograph shows prominent central markings, fluid in lung fissures and the occasional small pleural effusion.

2. E. Transposition of the great arteries

Transposition of the great arteries (TGA) is the most common cyanotic heart lesion to present in the newborn period. The aorta arises from the right ventricle, and the pulmonary artery arises from the left ventricle. This results in deoxygenated blood returning to the right heart and being pumped out to the body, while well-oxygenated blood returning from the lungs enters the left heart and is pumped back to the lungs. Without mixing of the two circulations, death can quickly occur. Initial medical management therefore involves the administration of prostaglandin E_1 to maintain ductal patency.

3. G. Neonatal abstinence syndrome

This is classical methadone withdrawal (also referred to as neonatal abstinence syndrome, or NAS). Symptoms of methadone withdrawal typically appear within 48–72 hours, but may not appear for up to 3 weeks. Signs of neonatal abstinence syndrome due to opiates include hyperirritability, gastrointestinal dysfunction, respiratory distress and vague autonomic symptoms (e.g. yawning, sneezing, mottling and fever). Tremors and jittery movements, high-pitched cries, increased muscle tone and irritability are also common, and reflexes may be exaggerated. Loose stools are common as well, leading to possible electrolyte imbalances and nappy rash.

4. L. Trisomy 18

Typical features of trisomy 18 (also known as Edwards' syndrome) include growth retardation, micrognathia (small mouth), clinodactyly, hypoplastic nails, overlapping fingers, rocker-bottom foot and cardiac abnormalities.

Most cases will die *in utero* or shortly after birth, with only 5% surviving longer than 1 year.

5. F. Neonatal lupus erythematosus

This is caused by transplacental passage of autoantibodies from a mother with systemic lupus erythematosus. Damage to the baby's cardiac conducting system results in congenital heart block. The mortality rate is approximately 20%, and most of the infants who survive require pacing.

2) K, I, H, A, D

1. K. Apnoea of prematurity

Apnoea of prematurity commonly occurs in newborns who are born before 34 weeks of pregnancy, and it increases in frequency and severity among the most prematurely born. In these newborns, the respiratory centre has not matured fully. As a result, the newborns may have repeated episodes of normal breathing that alternate with brief pauses in breathing. This is usually managed with caffeine therapy.

2. I. Necrotising enterocolitis

Necrotising enterocolitis (NEC) is a medical condition that is most commonly seen in premature infants, where portions of the bowel undergo necrosis. Initial symptoms include feeding intolerance and increased gastric aspirates, but this can progress to abdominal distension and bloody stools. A high index of suspicion is required to clinch this diagnosis early, as it can cause cardiovascular collapse, multi-organ failure and death.

3. H. Retinopathy of prematurity

Retinopathy of prematurity (ROP) is caused by the acute and chronic effects of oxygen toxicity on the developing blood vessels of the premature infant's retina. Excess oxygen causes vasoconstriction of the immature retinal vasculature in the first stage of this disease. The completely vascularised retina of the term infant is not susceptible to ROP. This condition is a leading cause of blindness in very-low-birthweight infants.

4. A. Patent ductus arteriosus

Patent ductus arteriosus (PDA) is treated with non-steroidal anti-inflammatory drugs such as indomethacin or ibuprofen. However, these drugs may also precipitate oliguria and renal failure.

5. D. Chronic lung disease

Chronic lung disease (CLD) is a clinical diagnosis defined by oxygen dependence at 36 weeks, and accompanied by characteristic radiological and clinical findings. In most cases it develops after ventilation for respiratory distress syndrome. The radiographic appearance of CLD may involve phases that are characterised initially by lung opacification and subsequently by the development of cysts accompanied by areas of over-distension and atelectasis, giving the lung a sponge-like appearance.

3) B, G, J, F, E

1. B. Physiological jaundice

Physiological jaundice is a common cause of hyperbilirubinaemia among newborns. It is a diagnosis of exclusion that is made after more serious causes of jaundice, such as metabolic disease, haemolysis and infection, have been ruled out. The clinical pattern of physiological jaundice is that of a mild to moderate jaundice that appears after 24 hours, being most significant at 3 days and resolving within 5 to 7 days. It should not be considered physiological if it is present on the first day of life, or if the bilirubin level increases rapidly, or if hepatosplenomegaly or anaemia are present.

2. G. Hydrops fetalis

Fetal hydrops is characterised by ascites, pleural and pericardial effusions and oedema. The risk of fetal death is high. Fetal hydrops can be caused by haemolytic disease of the newborn, characterised by haemolysis in a Rhesus-positive fetus whose Rhesus-negative mother has been sensitised to Rhesus antigens by blood from a Rhesus-positive fetus (typically from a previous pregnancy). This in turn causes fetal anaemia, heart failure and hypoalbuminaemia, which result in fetal hydrops.

3. J. ABO incompatibility

ABO blood group incompatibility with neonatal haemolysis only develops if the mother has IgG antibodies from previous exposure to A or B antigens. These IgG antibodies cross the placenta and affect the fetus or newborn. Usually ABO incompatibility only causes mild disease. With the declining incidence of Rhesus haemolytic disease (due to anti-D prophylaxis), ABO incompatibility has become the most common cause of neonatal hyperbilirubinaemia that requires therapy.

4. F. G6PD deficiency

Glucose-6-phosphate (G6PD) dehydrogenase deficiency is an X-linked inherited enzyme abnormality. G6PD helps to maintain glutathione in a reduced state, which in turn protects the red cells from oxidative injury. When G6PD is deficient, the red cells are at risk of haemolysis during periods of oxidative stress, or secondary to the administration of some drugs. Patients usually present with anaemia or jaundice, and can present in the neonatal period. G6PD deficiency is more common among African-Americans, but people of Mediterranean origin are also commonly affected.

5. E. Kernicterus

Kernicterus is damage to the brain of a newborn caused by increased levels of unconjugated bilirubin. High levels of unconjugated bilirubin may exceed the binding capacity of albumin. The excess bilirubin is then able to pass through the infant's blood–brain barrier, as it is lipid soluble. This results in deposition of bilirubin in the brain and irreversible damage. Neonates present with lethargy and hypotonia, which progress to irritability and seizures if not treated. Choreoathetoid cerebral palsy is a long-term sequela. Fortunately, kernicterus is rare, due to antenatal screening for Rhesus disease, and phototherapy.

4) C, F, I, K, D

1. C. Erb's palsy

This is a birth injury that affects the brachial plexus. It is the commonest form of this type of injury. The infant cannot abduct the arm at the shoulder, or externally rotate or supinate the forearm. The usual picture is one of painless adduction, internal rotation of the arm and pronation of the forearm. The Moro reflex is absent or abnormal on the involved side, and the hand grasp is intact.

2. F. Turner's syndrome

This is a characteristic description of Turner's syndrome (45 X). It occurs in 1 in 3200 births, and the signs in the neonatal period are usually subtle. The characteristic facial appearance includes low-set, mildly malformed ears, a triangular-shaped face, flattened nasal bridge and epicanthal folds. There may be webbing of the neck, with or without cystic hygroma, widely spaced nipples and puffiness of the hands and feet. Internal malformations include heart defects in 45% of cases (coartation of the aorta is the most common defect). Renal anomalies (e.g. horseshoe kidney and duplication of the collecting system) are seen in more than 50% of patients.

3. I. Cleft palate

An undiagnosed cleft palate can cause problems with establishing feeding. A cleft palate can be isolated or associated with a cleft lip. Babies often need special teats or occasionally may need nasogastric feeding. With the availability of increasingly detailed antenatal scans, many infants with cleft palates are detected antenatally, enabling appropriate counselling of the parents prior to delivery. Clefts are repaired by staged surgical repairs.

4. K. Cystic fibrosis

Meconium ileus causing gastrointestinal obstruction from a meconium plug is a common presenting symptom of cystic fibrosis, affecting 10% of patients. An abdominal radiograph would typically show multiple dilated small bowel loops. A barium enema shows a narrow, unused colon (microcolon). A sweat test (to detect cystic fibrosis) should be performed on all children with meconium ileus.

5. D. Congenital cataract

Failure to elicit a red reflex may be due to retinoblastoma or cataracts. If congenital cataracts are present, causes such as congenital infection or metabolic conditions should be ruled out.

2 Neurology and development

1) From the list of options below, please select the most likely diagnosis for each of the following scenarios concerning neurological problems that may occur in childhood. Each option may be used more than once.

   A. Cerebral palsy
   B. Infantile spasms
   C. Autism
   D. Asperger's syndrome
   E. Otits media
   F. Conductive deafness
   G. Paralytic strabismus
   H. Myoclonic jerks
   I. Plagiocephaly
   J. Brain tumour
   K. Non-paralytic strabismus
   L. Sensorineural deafness

   1. A 2-year-old, who had a difficult delivery, has been observed by nursery staff to be much clumsier than the other children. She also finds it difficult to copy shapes.

   2. A 4-year-old has presented to the GP surgery with a squint. There is a full range of movement in both eyes.

3. A 4-year-old boy has severely delayed speech and poor social interaction. He is obsessed with trains and will not go anywhere unless he has his toy train with him.

4. A 2-year-old girl is admitted with a high fever, irritability and a seizure. A lumbar puncture confirms meningitis. After she has been treated and discharged, nursery staff notice that she is more disruptive and she does not do what she is told.

5. A 2-year-old boy presents to the Accident and Emergency department. A few hours ago he became hot and flushed, his eyes rolled back, and he then became unconscious and stiff. The entire episode lasted about 5 minutes.

2) From the list of options below, please select the most likely diagnosis for each of the following scenarios, in all of which the patient presented with headache. Each option may be used more than once.

A. Vascular malformation
B. Migraine
C. Temporo-mandibular dysfunction
D. Subclinical seizure
E. Encephalitis
F. Craniopharyngioma
G. Hypertension
H. Intracerebral haemorrhage
I. Sinusitis
J. Benign intracranial hypertension
K. Tension headache
L. Head trauma

1. A 9-year-old girl presents with a paroxysmal, unilateral headache accompanied by nausea.

2. A 13-year-old girl presents with a bilateral, band-like headache that occurs on most days.

3. An 8-year-old boy presents with a history of a progressive headache over a period of a few months which is worse on lying down and first thing in the morning.

4. A 10-year-old boy presents with a headache that worsens on chewing.

5. A 6-year-old girl presents with a history of faltering growth and recurrent urinary tract infections that are accompanied by a chronic severe headache.

3) From the list of options below, please select the age at which most children reach the following developmental milestones. Each option may be used more than once.

A. Newborn
B. 6 weeks
C. 3 months
D. 6 months
E. 9 months
F. 12 months
G. 18 months
H. 2 years
I. 3 years
J. 4 years
K. 5 years
L. 10 years

1. A child can build a tower of six bricks.

2. A child can copy a circle.

3. A child can walk unsteadily.

4. A child can crawl.

5. A child can say a few words.

4) From the list of options below, please select the most likely diagnosis for each of the following scenarios, all of which involve children presenting with seizures. Each option may be used more than once.

A. Infantile spasms
B. Sturge–Weber disease
C. Breath-holding attacks
D. Simple partial seizure
E. Pseudoseizure
F. von-Hippel–Lindau disease
G. Reflex anoxic seizures
H. Complex partial seizure
I. Theophylline-induced seizures
J. Juvenile myoclonic epilepsy
K. Absence seizure
L. Tuberous sclerosis

1. A 7-year-old girl presents with episodes of abnormal movements involving the neck, face and extremities, associated with inappropriate speech, which last for about 10 seconds. She complains of 'feeling funny' just before an episode.

2. A 6-month-old boy presents with brief sudden contractions that result in flexion of the body. The attacks occur in clusters. He also appears to have developmental regression.

3. A 2-year-old girl has been experiencing sudden episodes of loss of consciousness. She appears very pale, becomes floppy and falls to the ground. Some fine twitching movements are observed, and the whole episode lasts about 20 seconds. The episodes are always triggered when she hurts herself.

4. A 12-year-old boy experiences involuntary muscle jerking while brushing his teeth each morning.

5. A 3 year-old child has left-sided seizures. A large right-sided facial naevus which has been present since birth is noted.

ANSWERS

1) A, K, C, L, E

1. A. Cerebral palsy

Mild cases of cerebral palsy may not always reach the specialist. If a child is clumsy, unable to march in step or finds it difficult to copy shapes, you should consider whether he or she may be in this 'missed diagnosis' group.

2. K. Non-paralytic strabismus

A squint (strabismus) is a misalignment of the eyes that results in the eyes not looking straight in the primary gaze. It is a common condition among children. A paralytic squint occurs when one eye does not move properly, due to a problem with either the muscle or the nerve. The eye movements are affected. In a non-paralytic squint the eyes can move normally individually, but when the two eyes are tested together there is a difference between them. Most squints in children are non-paralytic (concomitant).

3. C. Autism

Children with autism have severe and persistent difficulties in the following three broad areas:

- qualitative abnormalities in reciprocal social interaction with others
- abnormalities in patterns of communication
- a restricted and repetitive range of interests and activities.

Autism is fortunately a rare condition (about 1 in 1000), and it is more common in boys than in girls. Language problems are widespread, and most children do not develop early non-verbal means of communication. Children with Asperger's syndrome have similar problems to those with autism in relation to reciprocal social interactions and restricted social interests, but have relatively normal cognitive and language skills.

4. L. Sensorineural deafness

This is the most common form of permanent damage following meningitis. Damage can result both from the direct effect of the infection on the brain and from the body's response to the infection. The site of permanent hearing loss is almost always the cochlea. Damage usually occurs within the first couple of days of the illness. It is more commonly associated with pneumococcal meningitis. All children who have had meningitis should have a hearing test. Children with deafness will often have speech delay or appear to be disruptive (as they cannot hear what they are being asked to do).

5. E. Otitis media

This child has had a febrile convulsion secondary to an otitis media infection. Any illness that causes a fever can cause a febrile convulsion. Most occur with common illnesses, such as ear infections, coughs, colds, flu and other virus infections. Febrile convulsions are common in children between the ages of 6 months and 6 years. They are generally tonic–clonic seizures that are short-lasting.

2) B, K, F, C, G

1. B. Migraine

Migraine is a disorder characterised by paroxysmal, unilateral headache that is usually accompanied by visual disturbance (aura) and gastrointestinal symptoms such as nausea or abdominal pain. Occasionally there are unilateral sensory or motor symptoms.

2. K. Tension headache

This type of headache is usually of gradual onset, occurring frequently and in some cases on a daily basis. Tension headaches represent the majority of headaches in children, and can be due to factors such as stress or environmental triggers.

3. F. Craniopharyngioma

The key feature of increased intracranial pressure is a headache that worsens when lying down, as most types of headache (e.g. migraine) improve when lying down. In a child with such a history it is important to rule out a space-occupying lesion that is causing raised intracranial pressure.

4. C. Temporo-mandibular dysfunction

The term 'temporo-mandibular dysfunction' is used to describe a group of physical disorders that arise from an imbalance in the delicate working relationship of the jaw and skull with the muscles that move the jaw, as well as the nervous system associated with these systems. This imbalance results in muscle fatigue, spasm and/or joint dysfunction, and even changes in the teeth, which in turn cause a variety of symptoms, which vary from one person to another. Causes include habitual gum chewing or fingernail biting, dental problems and misalignment of the teeth (malocclusion), trauma and stress.

5. G. Hypertension

Most significant hypertension in childhood is due to renal causes. The history of faltering growth and recurrent urinary tract infections suggests an underlying history of chronic renal failure. Severe hypertension in children may cause headache, fatigue, blurred vision, epistaxis or facial nerve palsy.

3) H, I, F, E, F

1. H. 2 years

Children can usually build a tower of three bricks at 18 months, a tower of six bricks at 2 years, and a tower of eight bricks at 2½ years.

2. I. 3 years

A child can usually copy a circle at 3 years, a cross at 4 years, a square at 4½ years, and a triangle at 5 years.

3. F. 12 months

A child will usually start to walk at about 12–13 months of age.

4. E. 9 months

A child will usually crawl at about 9 months of age.

5. F. 12 months

A child will usually say 'mama', 'dada' and two to three other words by 12 months of age.

4) D, A, G, J, B

1. D. Simple partial seizure

This is a partial seizure because even though the child experiences an aura, she does not lose consciousness, and she verbalises during the episodes. Also there is no post-ictal period. If she had also experienced loss of consciousness, this would indicate a complex partial seizure.

2. A. Infantile spasms

Infantile spasms present in the first year of life, and the scenario demonstrates the typical history. The EEG shows disorganised activity known as hypsarrhythmia. Infants often have developmental arrest or regression. Infantile spasms may be idiopathic or symptomatic (caused by an underlying disease such as tuberous sclerosis).

3. G. Reflex anoxic seizure

This is a typical description of a reflex anoxic seizure. Usually episodes are triggered by a sudden unexpected painful stimulus, or occasionally by vomiting. Increased sensitivity of the vagus nerve causes severe bradycardia (or even brief asystole), leading to pallor and loss of consciousness. After the collapse the child may convulse. Recovery is spontaneous, and most children grow out of this condition.

4. J. Juvenile myoclonic epilepsy

Juvenile myoclonic epilepsy usually begins between the ages of 12 and 16 years. Patients note frequent myoclonic jerks on awakening, which abate during the course of the day. A few years later, early-morning tonic–clonic seizures develop in association with the myoclonus. The majority of cases respond to sodium valproate therapy, which is lifelong.

5. B. Sturge–Weber disease

Sturge–Weber disease is characterised by a facial port-wine naevus and an ipsilateral leptomeningeal angioma. This leads to ischaemic injury to the underlying cerebral cortex, and causes focal seizures and a hemiplegia on the contralateral side. It is also associated with some degree of mental retardation.

3 Immunology and infectious disease

QUESTIONS

1) From the list of options below, please select the most likely pathogen for each of the following scenarios, in all of which the patient presented with fever. Each option may be used more than once.

A. *Salmonella typhi*
B. *Mycobacterium kansasii*
C. Group A streptococci
D. Human immunodeficiency virus
E. *Plasmodium ovale*
F. *Haemophilus influenzae* type B
G. *Plasmodium falciparum*
H. *Mycobacterium tuberculosis*
I. Herpes simplex virus
J. Group B streptococci
K. Parainfluenza
L. *Staphylococcus aureus*

1. A 2-year-old girl develops a fever and stops moving her right arm. On examination she is found to have a swollen hot elbow. Movement of the joint is limited by pain.

2. The parents of a 2-year-old girl are worried because she has had a cold for the past 3 days, and she is now very hoarse and finds it difficult to breathe because of her barking cough, which is worse

at night. On examination you notice intermittent stridor. The child does not look toxic and her immunisations are up to date.

3. A 5-year-old child who has just returned from safari in Kenya develops symptoms of fever and rigors.

4. A 6-year-old boy has had high fevers and night sweats for 3 weeks. A chest radiograph reveals hilar lymphadenopathy.

5. A 5-year-old girl presents with a 3-day history of fever and sore throat. On examination she is found to have a red tongue and a generalised papular rash.

2) From the list of options below, please select the most likely diagnosis for each of the following scenarios concerning infections that affect the skin. Each option may be used more than once.

A. Infectious mononucleosis
B. Varicella zoster
C. Impetigo
D. Measles
E. Kawasaki's disease
F. Fifth disease
G. Meningitis
H. Roseola infantum
I. Erythema multiforme
J. Whooping cough
K. Lyme disease
L. Meningococcal sepsis

1. A 4-year-old boy presents with a 3-day history of a cough, coryzal symptoms and conjunctivitis. He then develops a high fever and a blotchy red maculo-papular rash which starts behind his ears and spreads to his face and then to the rest of his body.

2. A 9-year-old boy presents with ataxia and a vesicular rash that starts on his chest and gradually spreads out to his arms and legs in crops.

3. A 14-year-old girl presents with a florid maculo-papular rash after being treated by her GP for a sore throat and fever. On examination she is found to be mildly jaundiced.

4. A 5-year-old boy presents with a bright red eruption across both cheeks. His mother tells you that he has been 'a bit under the weather' for the past week.

5. A 7-year-old boy presents with a spreading purpuric rash, fever and signs of shock.

3) From the list of options below, please select the most likely diagnosis for each of the following scenarios concerning diseases that affect the immune system. Each option may be used more than once.

A. Systemic lupus erythematosus
B. Perforated bowel
C. Bacterial peritonitis
D. Nephritic syndrome
E. Human immunodeficiency virus
F. Coeliac disease
G. Appendicitis
H. Juvenile idiopathic arthritis
I. Influenza
J. Acquired immunodeficiency syndrome
K. Cow's milk intolerance
L. Severe combined immunodeficiency

1. A 2-month-old girl presents with a history of recurrent and atypical chest infections. Examination reveals severe wasting of the quadriceps and buttocks, with evidence of candidiasis in her mouth. Blood tests show undetectable levels of T cells, NK cells and immunoglobulins.

2. A 4-month-old girl presents with a history of recurrent infections over the past month. Her mother mentions that the child has also had persistent diarrhoea for the past 8 weeks and has poor weight gain. She is bottle fed and has not yet been weaned. Anti-endomysial and anti-glutamase antibodies are absent, but there is mild villous atrophy on jejunal biopsy.

3. A 3-year-old girl presents with a history of high fevers for 6 weeks, myalgia and joint pain. Examination reveals a salmon-pink maculo-papular rash, lymphadenopathy and hepatosplenomegaly. Her blood count shows a raised platelet count and leucocytosis.

4. A 4-month-old African girl with faltering growth and chronic diarrhoea develops recurrent chest infections and is diagnosed with *Pneumocystis carinii* pneumonia.

5. A 2-year-old child presents with fever, severe abdominal pain and a distended abdomen. On examination the child is found to be oedematous. Urine analysis reveals proteinuria, and blood investigations reveal leucocytosis with very low albumin levels.

4) From the list of options below, please select the most likely immunisation for each of the following statements concerning immunisations offered nationally. Each option may be used more than once.

A. DTP (diphtheria, tetanus, purtussis)
B. Yellow fever
C. Hib (*Haemophilus influenzae* type B)
D. IPV (polio)
E. Men C
F. MMR
G. BCG
H. PCV (pneumococcal conjugate vaccine)
I. Hepatitis B
J. HPV (human papillomavirus)
K. Hepatitis A
L. None of the above

1. Children with an allergy to eggs should be given this vaccine under hospital supervision.

2. Introduction of this vaccine has led to a 99% decrease in the incidence of acute epiglottitis.

3. Cerebral palsy is a contraindication for this immunisation.

4. A 12-year-old girl received this vaccine as part of an immunisation programme at school.

5. This live vaccine is given routinely in the UK at 13 months of age.

ANSWERS

1) L, K, G, H, C

1. L. *Staphylococcus aureus*

This child is likely to have septic arthritis, which is diagnosed by joint aspiration (usually under general anaesthetic). *Staphylococcus aureus* is the most common pathogen, although other causes include Group A streptococci and *Mycobacterium tuberculosis*.

2. K. Parainfluenza

The most likely diagnosis is croup (viral laryngotracheobronchitis), which accounts for over 95% of laryngotracheal infections. Parainfluenza viruses are the commonest cause, but other viruses, such as RSV and influenza, may cause this clinical scenario. It usually occurs between the ages of 6 months and 6 years. Typical features include a barking cough, fever, stridor, coryza and fever. An important differential diagnosis is acute epiglottitis, in which the child appears anxious and toxic, and often drools saliva. Without urgent treatment with intubation and intravenous antibiotics, deterioration and fatal airway obstruction may occur.

3. G. *Plasmodium falciparum*

Malaria is common in parts of sub-Saharan Africa. It is transmitted via the bite of the female *Anopheles* mosquito. *Plasmodium falciparum* is the most common pathogen found, and has the highest rates of complications and mortality. Other less common strains include *P. vivax*, *P. ovale* and *P. malariae*.

4. H. *Mycobacterium tuberculosis*

This child needs to be investigated for tuberculosis. Children may present with fever and malaise at the time of infection. However, if the condition goes unrecognised, they present later with complications such as progressive primary pulmonary TB, meningitis or septic arthritis. TB in children is usually acquired from an adult with open pulmonary TB, so contact tracing is important.

5. C. Group A streptococci

This is a case of scarlet fever. The initial symptoms are those of pharyngitis (sore throat). Toxins are released by Group A streptococci, which then cause a characteristic rash 2–3 days after the onset of a sore throat. The rash is typically a red punctate or papular rash, sometimes having the texture of course sandpaper. There may also be an associated strawberry tongue (white or red tongue with tiny red spots or papillae). After the rash has started to fade, there may be peeling of the skin on the hands.

2) D, B, A, F, L

1. D. Measles

Measles is an infection of the respiratory system caused by paramyxovirus, which is an RNA virus. Symptoms include fever, cough, runny nose, red eyes and a generalised maculo-papular erythematous rash which starts behind the ears and spreads sequentially to the face, arms, chest, abdomen, back and legs. Koplik's spots in the mouth are pathognomonic, but are usually only seen in the prodromal phase and have usually disappeared by the time the rash appears. The diagnosis can be confirmed by serology. Complications include interstitial pneumonitis, encephalomyelitis and subacute sclerosing panencephalitis.

2. B. Varicella zoster

Varicella zoster virus (chickenpox) is a common childhood condition. It is spread by respiratory droplets and characterised by a rash which occurs in crops for 3–5 days, starting on the head and trunk and progressing to the peripheries. It progresses from papular, to vesicular, to pustular in nature, and is often associated with pyrexia. Cerebellar ataxia is a benign complication of chickenpox, and is thought to be due to post-infection demyelination. Resolution occurs within 2–4 weeks.

3. A. Infectious mononucleosis

Infectious mononucleosis (glandular fever) is usually seen in older children, and is mainly caused by Epstein–Barr virus (EBV). It is characterised by fever, malaise, lymphadenopathy, tonsillitis and jaundice. Examination may also reveal hepatosplenomegaly. Ampicillin or amoxicillin should be avoided in these patients, as it causes a characteristic florid maculo-papular rash.

4. F. Fifth disease

Erythema infectiosum (also known as fifth disease or slapped cheek syndrome) is the most common illness caused by parvovirus, with a viraemic phase consisting of fever, malaise and myalgia, progressing to a characteristic reticular rash on the cheeks, trunk and limbs.

5. L. Meningococcal sepsis

Meningococcal sepsis is typified by purpuric skin lesions, which are irregular in size and outline and have a necrotic centre. Meningococcal sepsis (i.e. blood infection caused by *Neisseria meningitidis*) differs from meningitis (infection of the cerebrospinal fluid). Meningitis may be caused by a number of pathogens, including *N. meningitidis*, pneumococcus or

Haemophilus influenzae. Children with meningitis may present with fever, neck stiffness or photophobia, but younger infants and neonates often do not show these typical features.

3) L, K, H, J, C

1. L. Severe combined immunodeficiency

The most likely diagnosis is severe combined immunodeficiency (SCID). This is a genetic condition that causes severe defects in both cellular and humoral immunity. Both X-linked and autosomal recessive forms exist. It is characterised by recurrent infections which may involve opportunistic pathogens. The only curative option is bone-marrow transplantation.

2. K. Cow's milk intolerance

Cow's milk intolerance can present with chronic diarrhoea (with a protein-losing enteropathy) or enterocolitis (usually presenting with bloody diarrhoea). Biopsy of the small intestine typically shows villous atrophy with or without inflammatory colitis. Cow's milk intolerance can be treated by using lactose-free milks. In most cases, cow's milk is tolerated again by 2–3 years of age. Coeliac disease also causes villous atrophy, but is unlikely to present prior to weaning (as there would be no gluten in the infant's diet). Anti-endomysial antibodies are often positive in children with coeliac disease, but an IgA level should always be checked at the same time, as IgA deficiency causes a false-negative result (and is associated with coeliac disease).

3. H. Juvenile idiopathic arthritis

Juvenile idiopathic arthritis (JIA) is defined as a chronic arthritis that persists for a minimum of 6 consecutive weeks in one or more joints, commencing before the age of 16 years, after other causes have been actively excluded. Children may present with joint stiffness, swelling or pain. They may have systemic features such as rashes (typically salmon pink in colour), fevers, hepatosplenomegaly or malaise.

4. J. Acquired immunodeficiency syndrome

Human immunodeficiency virus (HIV) may be spread vertically to newborns antenatally, perinatally or postnatally. Risks can be decreased by the use of perinatal antiretroviral therapy and by avoiding breastfeeding. Infants who contract HIV in this way may present with faltering growth, diarrhoea or opportunistic infections. Unfortunately, this girl has developed *Pneumocystis carinii* pneumonia, which classifies her illness as acquired immunodeficiency syndrome (AIDS).

5. C. Bacterial peritonitis

Nephrotic syndrome is a triad of renal protein loss (proteinuria) which leads to hypoproteinaemia (mainly hypoalbuminaemia) and oedema. Hypercholesterolaemia is also a common finding, since the hypoproteinaemia stimulates hepatic lipoprotein synthesis. Immunocompromise arises due to immunoglobulin deficiency (immunoglobulins are proteins and are therefore also lost via the kidneys). Cases are therefore susceptible to infection, particularly with *Streptococcus pneumoniae* or *E. coli*, resulting in bacteraemia or spontaneous bacterial peritonitis.

4) L, C, L, J, F

1. L. None of the above

In the past there have been concerns that children with egg allergies would be at risk of an allergic reaction when receiving the MMR immunisation, but there is now good evidence that MMR can safely be given to children who have previously exhibited an anaphylactic reaction to egg. This is because the MMR is grown on chick cells, not egg whites or egg yolks. However, egg allergy is a contraindication to influenza or yellow fever vaccination.

2. C. Hib (*Haemophilus influenzae* type B)

Acute epiglottitis is a life-threatening emergency due to respiratory obstruction. There is intense swelling of the epiglottis and surrounding tissues, which is associated with septicaemia. The condition is almost exclusively caused by *Haemophilus influenzae* type B, which is why the Hib vaccine has been so effective.

3. L. None of the above

It is a common misconception that stable neurological conditions (such as cerebral palsy) are contraindications to immunisation. Some evolving neurological conditions may be grounds for deferring immunisation, but this should be discussed with the child's neurologist.

4. J. HPV (human papillomavirus)

All girls aged 12–13 years are now offered HPV immunisation to pro-tect them against HPV 16 and HPV 18, which cause cervical cancer. Schoolchildren (both boys and girls) aged between 13 and 18 years should also receive a diphtheria, tetanus and polio booster.

5. F. MMR

MMR is a live vaccine (to prevent measles, mumps and rubella) which is offered to infants at about 13 months of age. A booster is given as part of the pre-school boosters at around 3 years of age. The pneumococcus immunisation is also offered around 1 year of age, but this is not a live vaccine.

4 Gastroenterology and endocrinology

QUESTIONS

1) From the list of options below, please select the most likely diagnosis for each of the following scenarios concerning possible causes of faltering growth or short stature. Each option may be used more than once.

   A. Renal failure
   B. Trisomy 18
   C. Cortisol excess
   D. Kwashiorkor
   E. Monosomy 45 X
   F. Marasmus
   G. Familial short stature
   H. Edwards' syndrome
   I. Growth failure
   J. Klinefelter's syndrome
   K. Constitutional growth delay
   L. Deprivation dwarfism

   1. A 2-year-old girl who was born at term was subsequently diagnosed with infantile polycystic kidney disease. Her height has decreased from the 50th percentile at 6 months of age to below the 0.4th percentile currently.

2. An infant who is receiving treatment for West syndrome shows decreased linear growth.

3. An 11-year-old boy is being investigated for short stature. Both of his parents are of normal height. His bone age is delayed by more than two standard deviations from normal, and his growth rate remains in the lowest range of normal. All other investigations are normal.

4. A 2-year-old refugee has recently arrived in the UK and presents with gross oedema, muscle wasting, fatigue and multiple skin lesions.

5. A 4-year-old child is being investigated for short stature. She has missed several previous appointments and appears unkempt. Investigations are normal.

2) From the list of options below, please select the most likely diagnosis for each of the following scenarios concerning children who have had a change in their bowel movements. Each option may be used more than once.

A. Meconium ileus
B. Haemolysis
C. MALToma
D. Reye's syndrome
E. Colon cancer
F. Anal fissure
G. Hepatitis A
H. Lymphoma
I. Appendicitis
J. Meckel's diverticulum
K. Intussusception
L. Peptic ulceration

1. A 2-month-old boy presents with a history of intermittent acute abdominal pain accompanied by screaming and pallor, followed by a period of quietness. He has a centrally palpable sausage-shaped mass, and his mother reports that there has been blood and mucus in his stools.

2. A 4-year-old boy presents with a 2-day history of diarrhoea and vomiting, which his mother treated with aspirin. He is now hypoglycaemic with deranged liver function tests.

3. A 2-year-old girl presents after an episode of severe painless rectal bleeding. A technetium-99m pertechnetate scan shows a hot spot at the site of the ectopic mucosa.

4. A 4-year-old boy presents with non-specific abdominal pain and slightly loose stools. An X-ray shows a calcified faecolith.

5. A 5-year-old girl presents with a history of constipation and bleeding from the rectum when she has a bowel movement. She has experienced pain on passing stools for the past 2 weeks.

3) From the list of options below, please select the most likely test result for each of the following scenarios concerning presentation with poor growth in combination with other symptoms. Each option may be used more than once.

A. Reduced platelet count
B. Reducing substances in stool
C. Abnormal renal function
D. Stool rotavirus positive
E. Metabolic acidosis
F. Deranged liver function tests
G. High serum phenylalanine levels
H. Greatly elevated amylase activity
I. Metabolic alkalosis
J. High potassium levels
K. Delta F508 mutation
L. IgA anti-endomysial antibody positive

1. A 6-week-old boy, who has not regained his birth weight, presents with non-bilious projectile vomiting and dehydration. On examination, an olive-shaped mass is palpated in the upper abdomen.

2. A 2-year-old boy, who was born in India, arrived in the UK 2 weeks ago. He is very small for his age. He presents to the GP with a history of seizures. His skin appears hypopigmented and has a musty smell.

3. A 1-year-old British boy presents to his GP with a history of chronic weight loss, recurrent chest infections and breathing difficulties. His sweat test is positive.

4. An 8-month-old girl had a gastroenteritis infection 4 weeks ago. She has lost weight since then, and is experiencing continued symptoms of bloating, diarrhoea and irritability.

5. A 3-year-old girl presents with a history of chronic diarrhoea and weight loss. She is a fussy eater and does not like bread or pasta.

4) From the list of options below, please select the most likely cause for each of the following scenarios concerning childhood gastroenteritis. Each option may be used more than once.

A. Rotavirus
B. *Borrelia*
C. *Salmonella*
D. *Bacillus cereus*
E. *Shigella*
F. *Campylobacter*
G. *Yersinia*
H. *Mycobacterium*
I. *Leptospira*
J. *Giardia lamblia*
K. *Clostridium botulinum*
L. *E.coli*

1. A 13-year-old boy presents with nausea, vomiting, abdominal cramps and watery diarrhoea that began 2 hours after eating leftover takeaway for breakfast.

2. A 9-year-old girl has had diarrhoea for 3 weeks since arriving home from holiday. Stool microscopy showed cysts in the stool.

3. A 15-year-old boy presents with watery diarrhoea, vomiting and a descending paralysis.

4. A 16-year-old girl presents with fever, malaise, myalgia and bloody diarrhoea.

5. A 2-year-old girl presents with a 48-hour history of diarrhoea and vomiting. She is not dehydrated.

ANSWERS

1) A, C, K, D, L

1. A. Renal failure

The relationship between short stature and chronic renal disease in children is well documented, and is said to be due to a number of factors relating to the complex processing of vitamin D, and the role of the kidneys in the metabolism of growth hormone and osteogenesis. Infants who are diagnosed with infantile polycystic kidney disease tend to develop renal failure in the first few years of life. Short stature secondary to chronic renal failure is therefore the most likely answer in this case.

2. C. Cortisol excess

ACTH treatment is now either the first- or second-line treatment (depending on the physician) for West syndrome, and is also used in the management of some other forms of childhood epilepsy. Possible side-effects of this treatment include linear growth failure, weight gain (especially in the region of the trunk and face), hypertension, metabolic abnormalities, severe irritability, osteoporosis, sepsis and congestive heart failure. These side-effects occur due to stimulation of cortisol production by ACTH.

3. K. Constitutional growth delay

Constitutional growth delay (CGD) refers to a temporary delay in the skeletal growth and consequently the height of a child, with no other physical abnormalities causing the delay. Short stature may be the result of a growth pattern inherited from a parent (familial), or it may occur for no apparent reason (idiopathic). Typically growth slows down at some point during childhood, and eventually resumes at a normal rate. CGD is the most common cause of short stature and delayed puberty. As the bone age is delayed the final height is usually preserved – it just takes longer to be achieved (as although growth is slower, the epiphyses fuse later and so there are more growing years).

4. D. Kwashiorkor

Kwashiorkor or protein-dominant malnutrition occurs in the same parts of the world as marasmus, but is most commonly seen in older children, aged 2–4 years. At this age the next baby usually displaces the older sibling from the breast, and milk is replaced by a low-protein, starch-based diet. The child is listless, the face, limbs and abdomen swell, and the hair is sparse, dry and depigmented, especially on the legs. Diarrhoea is sometimes a feature. The distinction between the two forms of protein-dominant malnutrition is based on the presence (kwashiorkor) or absence (marasmus) of oedema. Marasmus is due to inadequate intake of protein and calories, whereas a child with kwashiorkor has inadequate protein intake but fair-to-normal calorie intake.

5. L. Deprivation dwarfism

Deprivation dwarfism is faltering growth in infants caused by emotional deprivation. It is important to rule out medical or dietary causes of faltering growth, as they often coexist in children who have suffered from abuse.

2) K, D, J, I, F

1. K. Intussusception

The symptoms are of intermittent acute abdominal pain with screaming and pallor followed by quietness. This describes colicky pain. There may also be a sausage-shaped mass that is palpable centrally, and emptiness of the right iliac fossa. In the case of a short history like that described above, the radiologist may confirm the diagnosis and the first-line treatment would be to reduce the intussusception with an air enema. If the intussusception is irreducible, surgery is necessary. The typical 'redcurrant-jelly' stool is caused by blood mixed with mucus. It is a late feature of the disease and indicates damage to the bowel.

2. D. Reye's syndrome

Occasionally, a child presents with decreased consciousness, hypoglycaemia and deranged liver function tests. This condition often follows a gastro-enteritis-type illness. It is related to aspirin, is known as Reye's syndrome, and is the reason aspirin is not often prescribed for children. Blood tests show very high ammonia levels. Death may occur due to cerebral oedema.

3. J. Meckel's diverticulum

A Meckel's diverticulum occurs in about 1 in 50 members of the population. Normally it causes no problems. It arises from the anti-mesenteric border of the terminal ileum, and is defined as the persistence of the intestinal end of the vitello-intestinal duct. The diverticulum or adjacent ileum occasionally contains gastric mucosa, and the acid produced by this ectopic mucosa causes ulceration and painless rectal bleeding which may be severe, and which most often presents during infancy. A technetium-99m pertechnetate scan will show a 'hot spot' at the site of the ectopic mucosa. These cases are managed by surgical excision of the ectopic mucosa.

4. I. Appendicitis

Up to the age of about 10 years, children find it difficult to describe and localise pain. Therefore the typical history of appendicitis pain that moves from the peri-umbilical region to the right iliac fossa may not be available. Regular review is the key to making a definitive diagnosis. Some children may have slightly loose stools due to irritation of the surrounding bowel. A raised white blood cell count with leucocytosis may be present. X-rays are not usually performed if appendicitis is suspected, but are sometimes required if other diagnoses are suspected. If an X-ray is performed, it may show signs of oedematous bowel, localised fluid level or the presence of a calcified faecolith.

5. F. Anal fissure

Anal fissure is common in children. It is caused by constipation, and leads to blood on the surface of stool and pain on defecation, which unfortunately exacerbates the constipation further. Management of anal fissures involves treating the constipation. Once the stool is soft, smaller and easier to pass, the fissure will heal spontaneously.

3) I, G, K, B, L

1. I. Metabolic alkalosis

This is typical of pyloric stenosis. Blood tests will reveal hypokalaemic, hypochloraemic metabolic alkalosis due to loss of gastric acid (which contains hydrochloric acid and potassium) as a result of persistent vomiting. The potassium concentration is decreased further by the release of aldosterone by the body in an attempt to compensate for the hypovolaemia due to the severe vomiting.

2. G. High serum phenylalanine levels

Phenylketonuria (PKU) is an autosomal recessive genetic disorder that is characterised by a deficiency in the hepatic enzyme phenylalanine hydroxylase (PAH). In the UK, cases are usually detected by the newborn screening programme. Untreated children are normal at birth, but they fail to attain early milestones, they develop microcephaly, and they show progressive impairment of cerebral function. Hyperactivity, EEG abnormalities and seizures and severe learning disabilities are the major problems later in life. A musty odour of skin, hair, sweat and urine (due to phenylacetate accumulation) and dermatitis are also observed. In contrast, affected children who are detected and treated are less likely to develop neurological problems or to have seizures and mental retardation, although such clinical disorders may still occur.

3. K. Delta F508 mutation

This infant has cystic fibrosis. This condition is caused by a mutation in the gene that encodes the cystic fibrosis transmembrane conductance regulator (CFTR). The most common mutation, ΔF508, is a deletion (Δ) of three nucleotides that results in loss of the amino acid phenylalanine (F) at the 508th position on the protein. This mutation accounts for two-thirds of CF cases worldwide. However, there are over 1400 other mutations that can produce CF.

4. B. Reducing substances in stool

This is a typical history of secondary lactase deficiency, which follows damage to the intestinal mucosa (e.g. acute viral or bacterial gastroenteritis), and resolves when the disease process is over and the intestinal mucosa heals. It is more common in children and especially in the developing world. The presence of reducing substances in the stool indicates that carbohydrates are not being absorbed.

5. L. IgA anti-endomysial antibody positive

This girl has coeliac disease. Some children will learn to avoid gluten-containing foods as these foods make them feel unwell. The diagnosis is confirmed by a small bowel biopsy while on a gluten-containing diet.

4) D, J, K, F, A

1. D. *Bacillus cereus*

Bacillus cereus is a Gram-positive, facultatively aerobic spore-forming bacterium whose cells are large rods. The emetic type of food poisoning is characterised by nausea and vomiting within 30 minutes to 6 hours after consumption of contaminated foods. Occasionally, abdominal cramps and diarrhoea may also occur. The duration of symptoms is generally less than 24 hours. The symptoms of this type of food-borne intoxication resemble those caused by *Staphylococcus aureus*.

2. J. *Giardia lamblia*

Giardia lamblia is a flagellated protozoan parasite that colonises and reproduces in the small intestine, causing giardiasis. Symptoms include persistent watery diarrhoea, malabsorption and faltering growth. Stools may show *Giardia lamblia* trophozoites or cysts. Remember that giardiasis is easily missed, and is an important cause of treatable diarrhoea. Symptoms of giardiasis can last for 2–6 weeks.

3. K. *Clostridium botulinum*

Clostridium botulinum is an anaerobic, Gram-positive, spore-forming rod that produces a potent neurotoxin. The onset of infection generally occurs 18–36 hours after exposure. Initial symptoms can include nausea, vomiting, abdominal cramps and diarrhoea. After the onset of neurological symptoms, constipation is typical. Dry mouth, blurred vision and diplopia are usually the earliest neurological symptoms. They are followed by dysphonia, dysarthria, dysphagia and peripheral muscle weakness. Symmetrical descending paralysis is characteristic of botulism. This contrasts with *Campylobacter* infection, which may precede Guillain–Barré syndrome and cause an ascending paralysis.

4. F. *Campylobacter*

Campylobacter infections cause ulcerations and oedema of the bowel wall, resulting in bloody diarrhoea. The incubation period is 2–7 days. Fever is often the initial symptom, with blood appearing 2–4 days after the onset of symptoms. *Campylobacter* can cause bacteraemia and sepsis, and is also associated with Guillain–Barré syndrome.

5. A. Rotavirus

Rotavirus is the most frequently identified cause of gastroenteritis in children under 5 years old worldwide. Virtually all children will suffer from diarrhoea and vomiting caused by rotavirus before they reach school age.

5 Cardiology and respiratory disease

QUESTIONS

1) From the list of options below, please select the most likely diagnosis for each of the following scenarios concerning cardiac disorders in paediatric patients. Each option may be used more than once.

   A. Transposition of the great arteries
   B. Physiological murmur
   C. Tetralogy of Fallot
   D. Ventricular septal defect
   E. Hypoplastic left heart
   F. Patent ductus arteriosus
   G. Aortic stenosis
   H. Atrial septal defect
   I. Duct-dependent coarctation of the aorta
   J. Persistent pulmonary hypertension
   K. Eisenmenger's syndrome
   L. Hypoplastic right heart

   1. An 8-year-old girl who is fit and well has been found to have an ejection systolic murmur of uniform intensity and brief duration. This murmur is intensified by fever, excitement and exercise. It varies in quality when she is examined lying down compared with sitting up.

2. A 6-week-old boy, who was born following a normal vaginal delivery weighing 3 kg, is being investigated for faltering growth, breathlessness and sweating on feeding. On examination he is tachycardic and tachypnoeic, and he has a parasternal thrill and a loud pansystolic murmur at the lower left sternal edge. He also has hepatomegaly.

3. During a routine newborn 'baby check' examination, a newborn boy was found to have absent femoral pulses and markedly higher blood pressure recordings in his arms than in his legs.

4. A 3-month-old boy was brought to the Accident and Emergency department when his parents noticed that he was becoming 'blue' on crying. Examination revealed a loud pansystolic murmur, and a chest radiograph showed a boot-shaped heart.

5. A newborn girl with tachypnoea and a high oxygen requirement has a loud second heart sound.

2) From the list of options below, please select the most appropriate first-line management for each of the following scenarios concerning cardiac conditions. Each option may be used more than once.

A. Heart transplantation
B. Antibiotic therapy
C. No intervention needed
D. Transvenous catheter balloon dilatation
E. Naloxone
F. Surgical closure
G. Immersion of the face in ice-cold water
H. Indomethacin infusion
I. Artificial ventilation
J. Prostaglandin infusion
K. Modified Blalock–Taussig (BT) shunt
L. Balloon atrial septostomy

1. A 5-year-old girl with a history of a previously corrected coarctation of the aorta presents with a history of recurrent fevers and a temperature of 39°C. Examination reveals that she has splinter haemorrhages of her nails and an erythematous rash on the palms of her hands.

2. A previously well 6-month-old boy presents with difficulty in feeding and breathlessness. On examination he has a pulse rate of 280 beats per minute.

3. A newborn girl developed cyanosis within the first few hours of life. An echocardiogram confirms that there are two separate parallel circuits.

4. A newborn boy who has been diagnosed with tetralogy of Fallot remains significantly cyanosed and is currently receiving a prostaglandin infusion.

5. A newborn boy is commenced on prostaglandin treatment for complex duct-dependent cardiac disease. He has pauses in his breathing, and a blood gas analysis shows hypercapnoea.

3) From the list of options below, please select the most likely diagnosis for each of the following scenarios concerning respiratory conditions. Each option may be used more than once.

A. Upper respiratory tract infection
B. Asthma
C. Inhaled foreign body
D. Acute epiglottitis
E. Tonsillitis
F. Croup
G. Bronchiolitis
H. Pertussis
I. Bronchiectasis
J. Bronchitis
K. Subglottic stenosis
L. Laryngomalacia

1. A 4-year-old boy who had missed some of his recommended vaccinations presented to the Accident and Emergency department with a fever and a sore throat. On examination he was drooling, sitting still and upright with an open mouth, with a soft inspiratory stridor. He looked scared.

2. A 1-year-old girl presented with a short history of coryza with paroxysmal spasmodic coughing which often resulted in the child vomiting. Staff on arrival noted an inspiratory whoop.

3. A 7-month-old ex-premature boy presented with a 2-day history of a sharp dry cough, coryza and difficulty in feeding. A chest radiograph revealed hyperinflation of the lungs and flattening of the diaphragm.

4. A 5-year-old boy with a history of recurrent chest infections has been admitted to hospital with increasing shortness of breath, night-time cough and wheeze.

5. A 2-year-old boy was playing with his older brother and had a sudden-onset shortness of breath. He appeared well and was playing when examined. However, auscultation revealed decreased air entry and wheeze on the right side of his chest.

4) From the list of options below, please select the most appropriate investigation for obtaining a definitive diagnosis for each of the following scenarios concerning respiratory illnesses. Each option may be used more than once.

A. Peak expiratory flow rate (PEFR)
B. Chest X-ray
C. Oxygen saturations
D. Hearing test
E. Barium swallow
F. Bronchoscopy
G. Per-nasal swab
H. Mantoux test
I. Sputum culture
J. Naso-pharyngeal aspirate
K. Sweat test
L. Throat swab

1. A 12-year-old boy has been on holiday visiting his family in Asia. After his arrival home he has a persistent productive cough and cervical lymphadenopathy.

2. A 6-month-old boy presents with tachypnoea. He has crackles and wheeze bilaterally on auscultation.

3. A 2-year-old girl presents with a history of choking on a peanut.

4. A 6-month-old girl is well and is gaining weight and height along the 50th percentile. Her parents report that she has been making an intermittent squeaky noise when breathing in. It has been present since birth and is worse on crying.

5. A 1-year-old boy presents with a history of faltering growth, chronic diarrhoea and recurrent chest infections.

ANSWERS

1) B, D, I, C, J

1. B. Physiological murmur

Innocent (also known as physiological, benign or functional) murmurs are present at some point in approximately 30% of children. This type of murmur arises due to the rapid flow and turbulence of blood in the great vessels and across normal heart valves. Innocent heart murmurs are characteristically asymptomatic, soft systolic murmurs. They may vary with change in posture or head position and respiration, and they are accentuated by increased cardiac output (e.g. due to fever, exercise or anaemia). There should be no radiation or parasternal thrill.

2. D. Ventricular septal defect

Ventricular septal defect is the most common congenital heart disease, occurring in approximately 2 in 1000 live births. Typical signs include a pansystolic murmur over the left lower sternal edge with or without a parasternal thrill. The murmur is caused by shunting of blood from the left to the right ventricle. If it is not treated, this can lead to heart failure (as in this case) during the neonatal period, or when the patient is older it may cause pulmonary hypertension and eventually Eisenmenger's syndrome. The majority of small defects close spontaneously, but larger defects may require surgical closure.

3. I. Duct-dependent coarctation of the aorta

Coarctation of the aorta is an outflow tract obstruction that occurs in a region where the thoracic aorta is constricted. In duct-dependent (obstructive) coarctation of the aorta, ductal tissue encircles the aorta and causes an obstruction as the duct closes. Signs can be picked up on routine examination, with a higher blood pressure in the upper limbs than in the lower limbs, or with poor or absent femoral pulses. A murmur may not be heard. If the condition is missed, the child may present with symptoms of heart failure or circulatory collapse. Non-obstructive coarctation of the aorta usually presents later in childhood or in adulthood, or is picked up on routine clinical examination. Signs include an ejection systolic murmur at the upper sternal edge, and hypertension in the right arm.

4. C. Tetralogy of Fallot

Tetralogy of Fallot is the most common cyanotic heart disease. It has four cardinal anatomical features, namely large ventricular septal defect (VSD), an overriding aorta, right ventricular hypertrophy and right ventricular outflow tract obstruction. The right ventricular outflow tract obstruction restricts blood flow to the lungs and leads to right ventricular hypertrophy with a right-to-left shunt through the VSD, resulting in cyanosis. This cyanosis typically becomes evident at 3–6 months of age, and is usually worse during exertion and crying. During these episodes of cyanosis the child may 'squat', which increases pulmonary blood flow and relieves their symptoms for a short while. The more severe the pulmonary stenosis, the earlier the presentation with cyanosis occurs.

5. J. Persistent pulmonary hypertension

Persistent pulmonary hypertension is when the systolic pulmonary artery pressure is higher than 50% of the systemic systolic pressure. It can be primary or secondary to another cause (e.g. meconium aspiration or hypoxia). Signs include respiratory distress and a loud second heart sound.

2) B, G, J, K, I

1. B. Antibiotic therapy

This is likely to be infective bacterial endocarditis, and it needs to be treated with intravenous antibiotics. It is usually caused by streptococcal infection introduced during minor procedures such as dental work, and is more common in patients who have had previous cardiac surgery. The presenting features are those of sepsis together with splinter haemorrhages, tender nodules on the fingers and toes (Osler's nodes), and changing heart murmurs. Even when treated with antibiotics, the mortality rate may be as high as 20%, and many cases have complications, including heart failure and systemic emboli, which cause brain abscess or stroke.

2. G. Immersion of the face in ice-cold water

This infant is likely to have a supraventricular tachycardia (SVT), which can be treated by plunging the baby's head into a bath of ice-cold water. It can also be treated by vagal stimulation or by administering IV adenosine. If the SVT continues, cardioversion may be necessary. SVT is the most common arrhythmia seen in childhood, and its causes are mostly due to re-entry within the atrioventricular node. It can be associated with Wolf–Parkinson–White pre-excitation syndrome, due to an abnormal re-entry circuit and an accessory conduction pathway in the heart.

3. J. Prostaglandin infusion

This is transposition of the great arteries, which is a cyanotic congenital heart disease in which there are two separate parallel circuits. The systemic venous blood passing through the right side of the heart returns directly to the systemic circulation via a connecting aorta. Pulmonary venous blood returns to the left side of the heart and is returned to the pulmonary circulation. This condition is not compatible with life unless there is another cardiac defect, such as an atrial septal defect (ASD), a ventricular septal defect (VSD) or a patent ductus arteriosus (PDA), to allow the mixing of the blood between the two circuits. Management is needed urgently, and prostaglandins are given to maintain the patency of the ductus arteriosus, which allows the circulations to mix. A balloon atrial septostomy (to make a hole between the right and left atria) may be required to allow further mixing of blood on a temporary basis. The corrective operation is an arterial switch, which is usually required within 2 weeks.

4. K. Modified Blalock–Taussig (BT) shunt

The management of tetralogy of Fallot requires initial medical treatment with prostaglandin infusion. However, ultimately surgery is required and the initial step is a modified Blalock–Taussig shunt to maintain pulmonary blood flow and oxygenation by creating a shunt between the subclavian and pulmonary arteries.

5. I. Artificial ventilation

Apnoeas (pauses in the breathing) that require intubation and ventilation are a well-known side-effect of prostaglandin therapy. Neonates on prostaglandin infusions should be monitored closely for apnoeas and respiratory insufficiency. This neonate has hypercapnoea and apnoeas, so ventilation is indicated.

3) D, H, G, B, C

1. D. Acute epiglottitis

Acute epiglottitis is a life-threatening emergency and is a rare cause of acute upper airway obstruction. It is due to *Haemophilus influenzae* type B, and is now rare due to the introduction of the Hib vaccine at 2, 3 and 4 months of age (UK schedule). The onset is usually very acute and the child is usually febrile, drooling and toxic, with a soft cough and a soft inspiratory stridor (due to swelling of the epiglottis, which causes upper airway obstruction). An anaesthetist should be involved in the management of this condition, and it is important not to upset the child or to attempt to examine them in a supine position or with an ENT examination, as this could compromise the airway. The protocol of Airway, Breathing and Circulation should be adhered to (usually the child is intubated), and IV antibiotics should be started.

Note: Stridor is an inspiratory noise caused by air passing through a narrowed larynx or trachea. It differs from wheeze, which is an expiratory noise.

2. H. Pertussis

Whooping cough is caused by infection with *Bordetella pertussis*. This causes paroxysmal coughing followed by an inspiratory whoop (although the whooping may not be present in younger infants). Blood investigation typically shows lymphocytosis, and a per-nasal swab confirms the diagnosis. Management is supportive with oxygen therapy and isolation, as it is a contagious condition, with endemics occurring every few years. Erythromycin can be given to reduce the infectivity to others, but it does not alter the course of the illness.

3. G. Bronchiolitis

Bronchiolitis is the commonest respiratory condition in infancy. Around 90% of cases are aged 1–9 months, and respiratory syncytial virus (RSV) is the causative agent in the majority of cases. Children with congenital heart disease, immunodeficiency and chronic lung disease of prematurity are at increased risk of this condition. Infants present with coryzal symptoms and a dry cough, which can lead to difficulties with breathing and feeding. Severe cases may have apnoeas and require ventilation. Typical signs include those of respiratory distress (e.g. recession, nasal flaring, head bobbing, tracheal tug), and auscultation reveals fine end-inspiratory crackles and expiratory wheeze. The liver may be displaced downward due to lung hyperinflation. Management is supportive, and oxygen therapy and nasogastric feeds or intravenous fluids are required in some cases.

4. B. Asthma

Asthma is a condition of chronic airway inflammation, airway hyperactivity and reversible airway obstruction. It affects 10–15% of the school-age population, and is the cause of 10–20% of all acute hospital admissions. It can present subtly with a night-time cough, or with a full-blown exacerbation. In the early stages it can often be misdiagnosed as recurrent chest infections. There is usually a family history of atopic illnesses.

5. C. Inhaled foreign body

It is likely that this child has inhaled a foreign body such as a small toy. An inhaled foreign body may present with coughing and choking, stridor, wheeze, respiratory distress or recurrent pneumonia. Signs may include wheeze or decreased air entry on one side of the chest. Recognition and removal (usually by bronchoscopy) are essential in order to avoid further complications, such as pneumonia or bronchiectasis.

4) I, J, F, F, K

1. I. Sputum culture

This child is likely to have tuberculosis. A Mantoux test and a chest radiograph would certainly be helpful, but if the child has a productive cough then sputum microscopy for acid-fast bacilli (AFB) and culture would be more likely to give a definitive result. In younger children, early-morning gastric washings can be used to look for AFB, as these children often swallow their sputum.

2. J. Naso-pharyngeal aspirate

Naso-pharyngeal aspirate is the investigation of choice for diagnosing bronchiolitis. Respiratory syncytial virus (RSV) is the commonest causative agent, but other viruses, such as influenza, parainfluenza or adenovirus, may also be causative, and a naso-pharyngeal aspirate can determine which virus is present.

3. F. Bronchoscopy

A chest radiograph may be useful, is often performed as a first-line investigation, and may show the foreign body or signs of hyperinflation or collapse. However, a definitive diagnosis is more likely to be made during bronchoscopy (especially if the object is not radio-opaque), which is usually performed under general anaesthesia. Treatment can also occur during bronchoscopy, as the foreign body can be removed during this procedure.

4. F. Bronchoscopy

This child most probably has laryngomalacia (floppy larynx). This condition causes stridor, which is variable but present from birth. The cartilaginous parts of the larynx and trachea are less firm than usual, and partly obstruct the airway on inspiration. It is a benign condition and usually resolves by 2 years of age. Usually the diagnosis is made clinically (to avoid invasive and unnecessary tests), but if the condition is persistent a bronchoscopy would confirm the diagnosis (and, more importantly, would rule out other more serious diagnoses).

5. K. Sweat test

This child may have cystic fibrosis. Infants may present with faltering growth due to increased energy needs and chronic malabsorption resulting from pancreatic insufficiency (which causes diarrhoea). The most appropriate test on the list is a sweat test, although DNA analysis can also be performed.

6 Orthopaedics and rheumatology

QUESTIONS

1) From the list of options below, please select the most appropriate form of management for each of the following scenarios concerning limb problems that may present in childhood. Each option may be used more than once.

A. Osteotomy
B. Oral steroid therapy
C. Abduction splint or harness
D. Arthroplasty
E. Physiotherapy
F. Immobilisation with collar and cuff
G. Traction
H. Physiotherapy and bisphosphonates
I. Oral antibiotics
J. Intravenous antibiotics
K. Non-steroidal anti-inflammatory drugs
L. Pin fixation

1. A 6-week-old baby girl was observed to have asymmetrical skin folds on her thighs. Ortolani's test was positive and an ultrasound scan confirmed the diagnosis.

2. A 7-year-old boy who is recovering from an episode of flu presents with a limp and has pain in his right hip on movement only.

He appears well and has normal inflammatory markers. A small joint effusion is visualised on ultrasound.

3. A 5-year-old boy presents with unilateral hip pain. His X-ray reveals increased density of the femoral head.

4. A 14-year-old boy presents with hip pain and restricted abduction following minor trauma while playing football. His diagnosis is confirmed by X-ray.

5. A newborn baby sustains fractures to her clavicle and humerus during an untraumatic delivery. She is observed to have blue sclera.

2) From the list of options below, please select the most likely diagnosis for each of the following scenarios concerning musculoskeletal deformities that may present in childhood. Each option may be used more than once.

A. Talipes equinovarus
B. Osteogenesis imperfecta
C. Skeletal dysplasia
D. Neurofibromatosis type 1
E. Kyphosis
F. Pes planus
G. Genu varum
H. Neurofibromatosis type 2
I. Positional talipes
J. Vitamin D deficiency
K. Friedreich's ataxia
L. Talipes calcaneovalgus

1. An 11-year-old girl presents with multiple brown spots on her back and a marked scoliosis.

2. A 9-year-old girl with a background of diabetes presents with a high arched painful foot.

3. A newborn boy presents with mild foot inversion which can be corrected to the neutral position by passive manipulation.

4. A 2-week-old girl's foot is noted to be supinated and inverted. It cannot be corrected by passive manipulation.

5. A 12-year-old boy presents with knock-knees and lethargy.

3) From the list of options below, please select the most likely causative agent for each of the following scenarios concerning patients with joint pain and other associated features. Each option may be used more than once.

A. *Staphyloccocus aureus*
B. *Mycoplasma*
C. *Campylobacter jejuni*
D. Varicella zoster virus
E. Group A streptococcus
F. *Escherichia coli*
G. *Haemophilus influenzae*
H. Group B streptococcus
I. *Borrelia afzelii*
J. *Clostridium difficile*
K. *Chlamydia trachomatis*
L. *Mycobacterium tuberculosis*

1. A 9-year-old girl presents with joint pain, headache, muscle soreness, fever and malaise. She also has a circular, outwardly expanding rash with target lesions.

2. A 16-year-old girl who is on the oral contraceptive pill presents with joint pain, dysuria, increased urinary frequency, fever, sore eyes and abdominal pain.

3. A 5-year-old boy presents with joint pain and fever. He has sub-cutaneous nodules on the back of his wrist and the outside of his elbows, and a widespread rash. He also has raised inflammatory markers and an abnormal ECG.

4. An 18-month-old baby presents with fever, a hot erythematous swollen knee and decreased range of movement.

5. A 9-year-old boy presents with joint pain, bloody diarrhoea, abdominal pain and vomiting. He was treated with antibiotics.

4) From the list of options below, please select the most likely diagnosis for each of the following scenarios concerning rheumatological problems and their differential diagnoses that may present in childhood. Each option may be used more than once.

A. Ankylosing spondylitis
B. Rheumatic fever
C. Pauciarticular juvenile idiopathic arthritis
D. Osgood–Schlatter disease
E. Kawasaki disease
F. Septic arthritis
G. Still's disease
H. Osteoid osteoma
I. Juvenile psoriatic arthritis
J. Torticollis
K. Scheuermann's disease
L. Osteopetrosis

1. A 13-year-old male footballer presents with knee pain.

2. A 6-year-old boy presents with fever, anorexia, dactylitis, nail pitting, a dry scaly rash and joint pain.

3. A 14-year-old boy presents with an increased kyphosis and lumbar back pain. His X-ray suggests osteochondrosis of the thoracic vertebrae.

4. A 5-year-old with a history of long-standing fever, swollen feet, an erythematous rash, cervical lymphadenopathy, red lips and conjunctivitis is now being treated in the Paediatric Intensive-Care Unit after suffering a myocardial infarction.

5. A 3-year-old girl presents with a high fever, malaise and persistent swelling of the knee, ankle, wrist and small joints of the hands and feet. She has hepatomegaly and raised inflammatory markers.

ANSWERS

1) C, K, E, L, H

1. C. Abduction splint or harness

Asymmetrical skin folds, limited abduction of the hips and apparent leg shortening are classic clinical features of developmental dysplasia of the hip with a dislocated hip. If diagnosed early, the infant is usually placed in a device that holds the hip in an abducted position, such as a Craig splint or a Pavlik harness, and progress is monitored by ultrasound or X-ray.

2. K. Non-steroidal anti-inflammatory drugs

Transient synovitis or irritable hip is the most common cause of acute hip pain in children aged 2–12 years. It commonly follows or presents accompanied by a viral infection. The inflammatory markers are usually normal or mildly elevated. There may be a small joint effusion detected on ultrasound. In contrast, septic arthritis typically presents with a markedly high temperature and inflammatory markers. The child would appear unwell and there would usually be pain at rest and they would not mobilise on the joint.

3. E. Physiotherapy

The age of this child, as well as the X-ray finding, points towards a diagnosis of Perthes' disease. The aim of treatment is to promote the healing process and to ensure that the femoral head remains well seated in the hip socket as it heals and regrows. In the past, children with Perthes' disease were treated with a plaster cast, a brace or surgery. However, it is now known that at least 50% of cases heal well without any treatment, particularly children aged 5 years or under, and milder cases. Most children with Perthes' disease are now treated conservatively with physiotherapy.

4. L. Pin fixation

Slipped upper femoral epiphysis (SUFE) is common at 10–15 years of age during the adolescent growth spurt. The presentation is fairly typical, with a limp or hip pain, and restricted internal rotation and abduction of the hip, and there may be a history of minor trauma. Management involves surgery, with pin fixation *in situ*.

5. H. Physiotherapy and bisphosphonates

This baby is likely to have osteogenesis imperfecta. Patients are treated with a combination of physiotherapy, bisphosphonates and physical aids.

Surgery may occasionally be required. Clavicle and occasionally humeral fractures may occur during traumatic vaginal deliveries. Such fractures are usually managed conservatively without the need to immobilise the arm.

2) D, K, I, A, J

1. D. Neurofibromatosis type 1

This is the most likely diagnosis. The brown spots in the question refer to the classical café au lait spots that are seen in neurofibromatosis. Scoliosis is also a common feature of neurofibromatosis.

2. K. Friedreich's ataxia

Friedreich's ataxia is an inherited disorder that causes progressive damage to the nervous system, resulting in symptoms such as gait disturbance, speech problems and heart disease. The diabetes, together with the high arched foot (pes cavus), are commonly recognised features of this condition. Other features include muscle weakness in the arms and legs, loss of coordination, visual impairment, hearing loss, slurred speech, curvature of the spine (scoliosis) and heart disease.

3. I. Positional talipes

This child has positional talipes as a result of his intrauterine position. The foot is of normal size, and the deformity is mild and can be corrected to the neutral position with passive manipulation.

4. A. Talipes equinovarus

Talipes equinovarus is a complex abnormality. The entire foot is inverted and the forefoot is abducted. The heel is in plantar flexion, and is rotated inwards. The affected foot is shorter and the calf muscles are thinner than normal. The position of the foot cannot be corrected to the normal position manually. Treatment is with serial casting initially.

5. J. Vitamin D deficiency

This child has rickets. This causes a softening of the bones, potentially leading to fractures and deformity. The predominant cause is vitamin D deficiency. The pattern of deformity varies according to the age of the child. Toddlers typically have bowed legs (genu varum), and older children typically have knock-knees (genu valgum) or 'windswept knees.'

3)   I, K, E, A, C

1. I. *Borrelia afzelii*

A rash that gradually expands over a period of days to weeks leaving central clearing (a bull's-eye or target lesion) is typical of Lyme disease, which is caused by bacteria belonging to the genus *Borrelia*. It is transmitted to humans by tick bites.

2. K. *Chlamydia trachomatis*

The most plausible explanation for these symptoms would be Reiter's syndrome. This is a triad of uveitis or conjunctivitis, arthritis and urethritis caused by a genito-urinary infection such as chlamydia. A urinary tract infection with *Escherichia coli* could cause fever, abdominal pain, dysuria and urinary frequency, but would be unlikely to cause joint pain or conjunctivitis.

3. E. Group A streptococcus

This collection of symptoms fulfils the revised Jones criteria for the diagnosis of rheumatic fever. The most common causative organism is Group A streptococcus.

4. A. *Staphyloccocus aureus*

This is septic arthritis until proven otherwise. The pathogen most commonly involved is *Staphylococcus aureus*.

5. C. *Campylobacter jejuni*

It is most likely to be campylobacter gastroenteritis causing a reactive arthritis. *Clostridium difficile* may cause bloody diarrhoea, but would only very rarely cause joint pain.

4) D, I, K, E, G

1. D. Osgood–Schlatter disease

Osgood–Schlatter disease is an inflammation of the growth plate at the tibial tuberosity. The condition occurs in active boys and girls aged 11–15 years, and coincides with growth spurts. The condition occurs more frequently in boys than in girls, and knee pain is usually the presenting symptom.

2. I. Juvenile psoriatic arthritis

This commonly involves the interphalangeal joints, and may also present with dactylitis (sausage-shaped swelling of the digits). The clinical criteria for diagnosis include arthritis and a typical psoriatic rash or arthritis plus three of the following: dactylitis, nail pitting, a psoriasis-like rash or a family history of psoriasis.

3. K. Scheuermann's disease

This is an osteochondritis of the thoracic vertebrae in adolescents that results in a fixed kyphosis. It is diagnosed on the basis of typical X-ray findings.

4. E. Kawasaki disease

This child meets the diagnostic criteria for Kawasaki disease, which is a systemic vasculitis that affects middle-sized arteries. This child has suffered its most serious effect, which is on the heart, where it can cause severe aneurysmal dilation and subsequent myocardial infarction, even in very young children. Around 20% of children who are affected have cardiovascular sequelae.

5. G. Still's disease

This is a presentation of systemic juvenile idiopathic arthritis or Still's disease. It usually affects young children. Clinical features include acute illness, aches and pains, lethargy, anorexia, weight loss and a salmon pink rash. There may also be lymphadenopathy and hepatosplenomegaly, and inflammatory markers are usually raised.

7 Haematology and oncology

QUESTIONS

1) From the list of options below, please select the most likely diagnosis for each of the following scenarios concerning childhood malignancies. Each option may be used more than once.

   A. Wilms' tumour
   B. Astrocytoma
   C. Non-Hodgkin's lymphoma
   D. Melanoma
   E. Ewing's sarcoma
   F. Osteosarcoma
   G. Acute lymphoblastic leukaemia
   H. Neuroblastoma
   I. Retinoblastoma
   J. Hepatic carcinoma
   K. Phaeochromocytoma
   L. Rhabdomyosarcoma

   1. A 3-year-old girl presents with abdominal pain, pallor and an abdominal mass. There are raised levels of catecholamines in her urine.

   2. A 15-year-old boy, who is a keen footballer, re-presents to the Accident and Emergency department with knee pain which had been reviewed 3 weeks previously. He is still suffering from pain

that wakes him up at night. Examination reveals a palpable hard mass at the lower end of his femur. A radiograph of his femur reveals a 'sunburst' appearance of bone formation.

3. A 4-year-old boy with aniridia, hypospadias and developmental delay is noted to have a large abdominal mass at a routine out-patient appointment.

4. A 2-year-old girl presents with unilateral leukocoria (loss of red reflex).

5. A 6-year-old girl presents with proptosis of her left eye.

2) From the list of options below, please select the most likely diagnosis for each of the following scenarios concerning conditions which affect the haematological system. Each option may be used more than once.

A. α-Thalassaemia
B. Aplastic anaemia
C. Hodgkin's lymphoma
D. Acute myeloid leukaemia
E. Acute lymphocytic leukaemia
F. G6PD deficiency
G. Non-Hodgkin's lymphoma
H. Iron-deficiency anaemia
I. Thrombotic thrombocytopenic purpura
J. Idiopathic thrombocytopenic purpura
K. Epstein–Barr virus
L. Sickle-cell anaemia

1. A 6-year-old girl presents to the hospital with a history of viral infection a few weeks ago, and has now developed petechiae, purpura and epistaxis. Blood tests reveal severe thrombocytopenia. She is otherwise well and is not pale.

2. A 12-year-old girl presents with fever, sore throat, enlarged lymph nodes, mild hepatomegaly and lethargy. Blood tests reveal an increased number of white blood cells and atypical lymphocytes.

3. A 15-year-old girl presents with a seizure. On CT scanning she is found to have a subdural haemorrhage. Blood tests reveal a pancytopenia. She is not jaundiced.

4. A 3-year-old girl presents to outpatients with mild developmental delay and pallor. She has pica (i.e. she eats non-food substances), but is otherwise well.

5. A 1-year-old boy from Angola develops mild shortness of breath and lethargy. Examination reveals that he is jaundiced. A full blood count reveals a microcytic, hypochromic anaemia.

3) From the list of options below, please select the most likely test finding for each of the following scenarios concerning conditions which affect the haematological system. Each option may be used more than once.

A. Absent factor VIII
B. Deficiency of collagen
C. Macrocytosis
D. Normocytic, normochromic anaemia
E. Elevated HbA2 and HbF
F. Raised copper levels
G. Haemolytic anaemia
H. Microcytosis
I. Decreased ferritin levels
J. Elevated haemoglobin and haematocrit
K. Pancytopenia
L. Elevated transferrin levels

1. A 5-year-old boy presents to the Accident and Emergency department shocked and unable to extend his right hip. He requires aggressive fluid resuscitation. He previously had to be admitted overnight after having a tooth removed.

2. A 16-year-old boy presents with a 1-month history of feeling generally unwell. He has developed a striking tan, but gives no history of sun exposure. Investigations reveal deranged liver function tests.

3. A 1-year-old girl from Iran presents with pallor, splenomegaly, bone abnormalities and lethargy due to severe anaemia.

4. A 7-year-old boy presents with increasing symptoms of breathlessness. He has also suffered from intermittent headaches. Examination reveals that his blood pressure is raised, and you note slight clubbing of his fingers and a systolic murmur. You immediately admit him to hospital.

5. A 12-year-old girl who has had a diagnosis of juvenile idiopathic arthritis since the age of 5 years presents with lethargy and pallor.

4) From the list of options below, please select the most appropriate treatment option for each of the following scenarios concerning haematological or oncological conditions that may present in childhood. Each option may be used more than once.

A. Recombinant factor VIII
B. Surgical excision
C. IV fluids and allopurinol
D. Bone-marrow transplant
E. Amphotericin
F. Splenectomy
G. Steroids
H. Desmopressin
I. IV fluids and analgesia
J. Radiotherapy
K. Chemotherapy
L. Recombinant factor IX

1. An 8-year-old boy presents with a large haematoma in his thigh after a fall, which despite all measures cannot be controlled. He is known to have Christmas disease.

2. A 4-year-old girl who is having chemotherapy for osteosarcoma presents with a fever of 39°C and neutropenia. She has been treated with two different combinations of broad-spectrum antibiotics for a total of 7 days, but still has a raised temperature.

3. A 3-year-old boy of African descent presents with a 1-day history of severe pain and swelling in both hands and feet. He cannot walk or play with his toys due to the pain. His sister has the same condition.

4. A 13-year-old girl suffers from severe menorrhagia and is told that she has a blood disorder which is causing her heavy periods. Investigations reveal a normal INR and APTT but a prolonged bleeding time.

5. A 10-year-old girl presents with spontaneous bruising and severe pallor. Investigations reveal anaemia, thrombocytopenia and a lymphocytosis of 50×10^9/l, with 80% blast cells seen on blood film.

ANSWERS

1) H, F, A, I, L

1. H. Neuroblastoma

Neuroblastoma is a common tumour of neural crest origin which may develop at any site of the sympathetic nervous system tissue, but most commonly arises in the abdomen. Abdominal neuroblastoma commonly presents as a hard, fixed abdominal mass that causes discomfort. Tumour markers are elevated in 95% of cases and help to confirm the diagnosis (i.e. elevated homovanillic acid (HVA) and vanillylmandelic acid (VMA) in the urine). Pathological diagnosis is made on the basis of biopsy of tumour tissue.

2. F. Osteosarcoma

Osteosarcoma is the most common primary malignant bone tumour in children and adolescents, followed by Ewing's sarcoma. The highest risk of development occurs during the adolescent growth spurt. Osteosarcoma presents with local pain and swelling at the site of the tumour, and there is often a history of injury. Radiography may reveal the classic 'sunburst' pattern, caused by periosteal reaction to the tumour. The above scenario could describe an osteosarcoma or a Ewing's sarcoma, but osteosarcoma is the most common and therefore the most likely diagnosis.

3. A. Wilms' tumour

Wilms' tumour accounts for most renal neoplasms in childhood. An important feature of Wilms' tumour is its association with congenital abnormalities such as hydrospadias, aniridia, organomegaly and mental retardation.

4. I. Retinoblastoma

Retinoblastoma classically presents with a white pupillary reflex (leukocoria). However, strabismus, pupil irregularity and hyphema (blood in the anterior chamber of the eye) are also features of this condition, the latter being indicative of advanced disease.

5. L. Rhabdomyosarcoma

Rhabdomyosarcoma is a tumour that is thought to originate from primitive muscle cells. It is the most common soft tissue sarcoma in children, and normally presents as an expanding soft tissue mass. It can present anywhere in the body, but does not affect bone. It has a wide variety of presentations, depending on the site involved. Generally it affects children under 15 years of age (patients aged 2–6 years tend to suffer from head, neck and genito-urinary tumours, and those aged 14–18 years tend to present with tumour in the extremities, trunk and paratesticular location). Orbital rhabdomyosarcoma may present with proptosis or a dysconjugate gaze.

2) J, K, B, H, L

1. J. Idiopathic thrombocytopenic purpura

Idiopathic thrombocytopenic purpura (ITP) is a disease characterised by platelet destruction. It commonly develops after a viral illness. Patients present with bruises or a petechial rash and have low platelet counts, with an otherwise normal blood count and film. Although life-threatening haemorrhage is uncommon, it can occur, and some children (< 1%) may present with intracranial haemorrhage. The disease usually resolves within 2–3 months without treatment. However, IV immunogloblins, steroids and platelet transfusions can be used. Splenectomy is considered in patients with chronic ITP (i.e. lasting for more than 6 months).

2. K. Epstein–Barr virus

Epstein–Barr virus (EBV) can commonly present with cervical lymphadenopathy, sore throat, hepatomegaly and anaemia. It is an important differential diagnosis for a simple viral or bacterial tonsillitis. Blood tests reveal lymphocytosis, which differentiates it from a bacterial infection (predominantly neutrophils).

3. B. Aplastic anaemia

In aplastic anaemia the haematopoietic elements of the bone marrow disappear, the marrow is replaced by fat, and there is a resulting pancytopenia. In developed countries, aplastic anaemia is usually idiopathic. Alternatively, it may follow the administration of certain drugs, or it may follow infections such as hepatitis or glandular fever.

4. H. Iron-deficiency anaemia

Iron-deficiency anaemia is the most likely option. It can cause developmental delay or mild learning difficulties at school. A blood test would show hypochromic microcytic anaemia, and ferritin levels would usually be low. Some children with iron-deficiency anaemia exhibit pica (the ingestion of non-food substances). This resolves with iron treatment.

5. L. Sickle-cell anaemia

Sickle-cell anaemia is caused by a mutation in the gene that encodes the beta chains of the haemoglobin molecule. This mutation results in the haemoglobin molecule becoming deformed or 'sickled' in shape (HbS). It is a genetic disease, which is inherited in a recessive fashion. In the UK it is screened for as part of the blood spot test that babies have when they are about 5 days old. However, children coming from other countries may not have been tested at birth and so may not present until they are symptomatic. Children commonly present with pallor, lethargy and mild jaundice. Sickle-cell anaemia commonly affects people of sub-Saharan African descent, and usually presents after the age of 6 months, when fetal haemoglobin levels decline and the HbS levels become clinically significant. Interestingly, heterozygotes have an increased resistance to malaria.

3) A, L, E, J, D

1. A. Absent factor VIII

This is a presentation of haemophilia A (absence of clotting factor VIII). Although most muscular haemorrhages are visible, patients can lose large volumes of blood into their iliopsoas muscle, presenting with hypovolaemic shock with only a vague area of referred pain in the groin. The bleed can be diagnosed clinically by the inability to extend the hip, but requires confirmation by ultrasound or CT. The recent admission may have been due to excessive bleeding after the tooth was removed, which suggests a possible bleeding disorder (children don't usually need to stay in hospital after a tooth extraction).

2. L. Elevated transferrin levels

Elevated serum transferrin, iron and ferritin levels are typical of haemochromatosis, as is the classic presenting triad of bronzed skin, cirrhosis and diabetes, the latter two symptoms occurring later in the disease course.

3. E. Elevated HbA2 and HbF

The diagnosis is beta thalassaemia major. It typically presents during the first few months of life, once the fetal haemoglobin (HbF) level has decreased. The HbF level decreases naturally after birth, and as it does so, the impact of beta-haemoglobin deficiency becomes apparent. In order to try to compensate, the overall levels of HbF remain higher than normal. The bone abnormalities and splenomegaly are due to extramedullary erythropoiesis.

4. J. Elevated haemoglobin and haematocrit

Elevated haemoglobin and haematocrit occur in polycythaemia. Primary polycythaemia is fairly rare. However, there are many causes of secondary polycythaemia. In this case, it was due to a previously undiagnosed VSD causing polycythaemia secondary to hypoxia.

5. D. Normocytic, normochromic anaemia

Some children with chronic diseases can develop normocytic, normochromic anaemia, known as *anaemia of chronic disease*. The ideal treatment for the anaemia involves successful treatment of the chronic disease. A full history and examination still need to be undertaken, and investigations should be performed to rule out any other possible cause of anaemia.

4) L, E, I, H, C

1. L. Recombinant factor IX

Christmas disease, also known as haemophilia B, is an inherited deficiency of factor IX. It is inherited in an X-linked manner. Haemophilia A is also an X-linked inherited disorder, which results in a deficiency of factor VIII. Each disease has varying degrees of severity depending on the quantity of each factor in the blood. Treatment of a severe bleed consists of infusion of the appropriate clotting factor.

2. E. Amphotericin

This case presented with neutropenic sepsis. This condition is treated initially with broad-spectrum antibiotics. However, in this case the patient was still pyrexial after 7 days of antibiotic treatment. Patients on chemotherapy are susceptible to fungal infection. Therefore if the pyrexia continues despite antibiotic therapy, antifungal agents such as amphotericin should be considered.

3. I. IV fluid and analgesia

This patient is presenting with a sickle-cell crisis. Young children are more likely to present with pain and swelling in the hands and feet, whereas older children and adults are more likely to present with pain in the long bones, back and abdomen. Sickle-cell crises occur when the sickled haemoglobin occludes small vessels, causing tissue infarction. Risk factors for a sickle crisis include dehydration, infection, hypoxia and acidosis. Treatment includes IV hydration and adequate analgesia, as well as treatment of any underlying infection if present.

4. H. Desmopressin

This patient has Von Willebrand's disease. This is an autosomal dominant condition which results in an abnormal, low or absent Von Willebrand factor (vWF). vWF is needed for platelet adhesion and stabilisation of factor VIII. Symptoms include bruising and mucosal bleeding (e.g. bleeding from the gums, epistaxis, menorrhagia). Tests reveal a prolonged bleeding time. Treatment depends on the levels of vWF in the blood. For mild disease, desmopressin is used, as this promotes the release of vWF from endothelium.

5. C. IV fluid and allopurinol

This is a presentation of acute lymphoblastic leukaemia. The child has a greatly elevated lymphocyte count, with a high percentage of blast cells observed. The child should be given IV fluids and allopurinol prior to chemotherapy or steroids in order to reduce the risk of tumour lysis syndrome. The latter is a serious metabolic complication associated with certain tumours, which causes acute renal failure and potentially death. If this child was to be given chemotherapy or steroids initially, this could induce or worsen tumour lysis syndrome.

8 Nephrology and urology

QUESTIONS

1) From the list of options below, please select the most appropriate investigation to perform next for each of the following scenarios concerning genito-urinary or renal problems that are encountered in neonates. Each option may be used more than once.

   A. Serum urea and creatinine
   B. Outpatient abdominal ultrasound scan
   C. DMSA
   D. Urgent MCUG
   E. Abdominal plain X-ray
   F. Urine multistick
   G. Routine MCUG
   H. Urine reducing substances
   I. Chromosomes
   J. Blood glucose
   K. MAG 3 scan
   L. None of the above

   1. A newborn baby has ambiguous genitalia identified shortly after birth.

   2. A newborn baby girl had antenatally diagnosed moderate unilateral renal pelvis dilatation.

   3. A newborn baby boy had antenatally diagnosed severe bilateral renal pelvis dilatation.

4. A 3-week-old girl has been admitted with a urinary tract infection associated with sepsis. She had an inpatient ultrasound scan which was normal.

5. A newborn boy has a unilateral undescended testicle.

2) From the list of options below, please select the investigation that is most likely to lead to a diagnosis for each of the following scenarios concerning patients who have had their urine checked with multi-sticks. Each option may be used more than once.

A. Serum albumin
B. Serum urea and creatinine
C. Abdominal X-ray
D. Paired serum and urine osmolality
E. Anti-streptolysin O titre
F. Blood glucose
G. Urine microscopy and culture
H. Stool culture
I. Full blood count and blood film
J. Abdominal ultrasound
K. Liver biopsy
L. Throat swab for culture

1. An 8-year-old girl presents with fever, dysuria and difficulty in passing urine. Urine multistick showed 3+ leukocytes and was positive for nitrites.

2. A 3-year-old boy with a recent onset of diarrhoea presents very unwell with pallor and a delayed capillary refill time. Urine multistick showed 2+ blood and 2+ protein.

3. A 7-year-old girl presents with polyuria and secondary nocturnal enuresis. Her urine multistick is normal, but you notice that her urine is very pale.

4. An 8-year-old girl, who recently had a throat infection, presents with dark urine. Her blood pressure is raised and her urine dipstick shows 3+ blood and 3+ protein.

5. A 3-year-old boy presents with swelling of his eyelids. Examination reveals that he has generalised oedema and ascites. His urine shows 3+ proteinuria.

3) From the list of options below, please select the most likely diagnosis for each of the following scenarios concerning patients who presented with biochemical disturbances. Each option may be used more than once.

   A. Fanconi's anaemia
   B. Bartter's syndrome
   C. Distal renal tubular acidosis
   D. Nephrogenic diabetes insipidus
   E. Metabolic bone disease of prematurity
   F. Vitamin D deficiency rickets
   G. Primary hypoparathyroidism
   H. Nephrotic syndrome
   I. X-linked hypophosphataemic rickets
   J. Pseudohypoparathyroidism
   K. Pseudo-Bartter's syndrome
   L. Proximal renal tubular acidosis

   1. A 12-month-old boy presents with faltering growth and swollen wrists. Wrist X-rays show cupping and fraying of the metaphyseal region. His blood test results are as follows:
      • ALP raised
      • phosphate low
      • calcium normal
      • PTH normal
      • 25-hydroxy vitamin D normal.

   2. A 4-year-old girl presents with genu valgum (knock-knee) deformity. Her blood test results are as follows:
      • ALP raised
      • phosphate low
      • calcium normal
      • PTH raised
      • 25-hydroxy vitamin D low.

   3. A 2-week-old boy with dysmorphic features presents with seizures and is found to have hypocalcaemia. His blood test results are as follows:
      • ALP normal
      • phosphate raised
      • calcium low

- PTH low
- 25-hydroxy vitamin D normal.

4. An 18-month-old boy presents with faltering growth and vomiting. His blood and urine test results are as follows:
   - serum potassium 3.0 mmol/l
   - serum pH 7.2
   - serum bicarbonate 15 mmol/l
   - serum CO_2 3.5 kPa
   - urine pH 5.0.

5. A 5-year-old boy presents with loin pain. His blood and urine test results are as follows:
   - serum potassium 3.0 mmol/l
   - serum pH 7.2
   - serum bicarbonate 15 mmol/l
   - serum CO_2 3.5 kPa
   - urine pH 7.0.

4) From the list of options below, please select the most appropriate management for each of the following scenarios concerning urological problems in children. Each option may be used more than once.

A. Desmopressin
B. Circumcision
C. Advise against circumcision
D. Enuresis alarm
E. Advise the use of incontinence pads
F. Ultrasound scan
G. Send swab for culture
H. Upper pole hemi-nephrectomy
I. Exploratory surgery
J. Course of oral antibiotics
K. Hernia repair
L. None of the above

1. A 3-year-old boy presents with a painful left testicle.

2. A newborn boy has a swelling of the left scrotal sac. The left testicle can be felt within the swelling. The swelling transilluminates.

3. A 5-year-old boy presents with a history of ballooning of the foreskin when he passes urine. He is now finding it difficult to pass urine. Examination reveals that he has a tight non-retractile foreskin and a tender palpable mass in the lower abdomen.

4. A 6-year-old girl with a duplex right kidney continues to have daytime and nocturnal enuresis. Her mother reports that the girl is constantly dribbling urine.

5. A newborn boy has a urethral meatus on the ventral surface of his penis.

ANSWERS

1) I, B, D, G, L

1. I. Chromosomes

It is important to check the chromosomes as soon as possible in babies with ambiguous genitalia. Families are keen to know the gender of their baby so that they can inform family members and choose a name. It is important that they do not register the birth of the baby until the gender is known, as it is difficult to change the register afterwards. Often an ultrasound scan is also arranged to look for intra-abdominal gonads, but checking the chromosomes is essential.

2. B. Outpatient abdominal ultrasound scan

Newborns with antenatally diagnosed renal pelvic dilatation should have an early neonatal scan to confirm the findings. The level of urgency depends on the severity of the dilatation, but an appointment can usually be arranged as an outpatient. If the neonatal scan demonstrates persistence of the renal pelvic dilatation, a micturating cysto-urethrogram (MCUG) is usually required to look for vesico-ureteric reflux. Infants should also be commenced on prophylactic antibiotics to prevent urinary infections.

3. D. Urgent MCUG

This baby probably has a posterior urethral valve. This is an abnormal congenital membrane in the posterior urethra, which causes partial obstruction of urine flow, as a consequence of which urine accumulates in the posterior urethra and bladder. An urgent inpatient MCUG test is needed to diagnose this. The MCUG would show a dilated posterior urethra and a dilated thick-walled bladder.

4. G. Routine MCUG

This baby has had a urine infection at an early age. Although her ultrasound scan was normal, she requires a routine MCUG to check for vesico-ureteric reflux. During the MCUG a catheter is passed into the bladder, and dye is then introduced into the catheter so that the outline of the bladder can be seen. When the patient micturates, the urine should leave the bladder via the urethra and should not go back up the ureters towards the kidneys – if it does so, this is diagnostic of vesico-ureteric reflux. The MCUG should not be performed soon after a urinary infection, as there is a risk of infection spreading to the kidneys as a result of the procedure.

5. L. None of the above

It is fairly common for baby boys to have unilateral undescended testicles when they are born. So long as the genitalia appear otherwise normal, simple reassurance of the parents is all that is needed. You should advise the parents to mention the condition at the baby's 6-week check so that it can be checked again. Usually the testicle will descend spontaneously. If it does not, it may require surgical correction at 6–12 months of age to reduce the risk of infertility and testicular cancer.

2) G, I, D, E, A

1. G. Urine microscopy and culture

This girl most probably has a lower urinary tract infection. She should have at least one urine sample sent for microscopy and culture. Most simple urinary infections can be treated with a course of oral antibiotics. Upper urinary tract infections (such as pyelonephritis) usually require intravenous antibiotics. A single urinary infection in an otherwise healthy 8-year-old would not require any follow-up or investigations.

2. I. Full blood count and blood film

This child has haemolytic uraemic syndrome, which is the commonest cause of acute renal failure in children. It is usually associated with diarrhoea (when it is referred to as D+ HUS), most commonly due to *E. coli* 0157, which produces verocytotoxin (also called Shiga toxin). The toxin is released in the gut and absorbed, causing endothelial damage that leads to microangiopathic haemolytic anaemia with thrombocytopenia and red blood cell fragmentation (detected on full blood count and blood film). The microangiopathy leads to patchy focal thrombosis and infarction, and causes renal failure (often requiring dialysis). Hence there may well be some renal impairment demonstrable by checking the serum urea and electrolytes, but a full blood count is more likely to provide the underlying diagnosis. A stool culture may show *E. coli* 0157, but this is likely to take several days to confirm, and a full blood count confirms the diagnosis more quickly.

3. D. Paired serum and urine osmolality

This child may have central diabetes insipidus. Patients with this condition have insufficient arginine vasopressin (AVP). AVP regulates the permeability of the luminal membrane of the collecting ducts. Low levels of AVP cause decreased permeability at the collecting ducts, which means that water cannot be reabsorbed and the urine is dilute. As a result, patients are at risk of becoming dehydrated, but with an intact thirst mechanism most children will drink copious amounts of water to try to maintain a normal serum osmolality. In this child, a normal urine multistix (i.e. absence of glycosuria) makes a diagnosis of diabetes mellitus unlikely.

4. E. Anti-streptolysin O titre

This child has acute post-streptococcal glomerulonephritis. Anti-streptolysin O titre (ASOT) tests for recent *Streptococcus* infection, which helps to confirm the diagnosis. Children typically present with reddish-brown (coca-cola-coloured) urine 10–14 days after a streptococcal throat or skin infection. A throat swab could also be taken, but it will be several days before the result is available, and often the infection will have resolved or been treated by the time of presentation. Complement levels should also be checked, and typically show reduced C3 but normal C4 levels.

5. A. Serum albumin

This boy has nephrotic syndrome. This is a triad of oedema, proteinuria and hypoalbuminaemia. It is almost always idiopathic in childhood, and it is usually steroid sensitive. In most cases, histology would show minimal change nephropathy, but biopsies are not required for most children.

3) I, F, G, L, C

1. I. X-linked hypophosphataemic rickets

In this condition, a mutation in the PEX gene on the X chromosome causes an isolated defect in phosphate reabsorption. This low rate of tubular reabsorption of phosphate results in hypophosphataemia, and therefore rickets develops. Typical radiological changes in rickets include cupping and fraying of the metaphyseal regions. Other features include delayed dentition. The normal 25-hydroxy vitamin D and PTH levels, together with a low phosphate level, provide the clue to the diagnosis.

2. F. Vitamin D deficiency rickets

This child has vitamin D deficiency leading to rickets. The low 25-hydroxy vitamin D level provides the clue to the diagnosis. This child requires a careful detailed history of diet and sun exposure. Rickets typically causes genu varum (bowed legs) in children under 2 years of age, and genu valgum (knock-knees) in children over 2 years of age.

3. G. Primary hypoparathyroidism

Low parathyroid hormone levels result in hyperphosphataemia and hypocalcaemia. The seizures are likely to be secondary to hypocalcaemia. In this case the hypoparathyroidism is likely to be due to Di George syndrome (congenital abnormality of the third and fourth brachial arches leading to hypoparathyroidism, absent thymus, dysmorphic features and congenital cardiac disease).

4. L. Proximal renal tubular acidosis

Proximal (type 2) renal tubular acidosis is caused when there is reduced proximal tubular reabsorption of bicarbonate. Normally 85% of the filtered bicarbonate is reabsorbed in the proximal tubule. The distal tubule cannot fully compensate for this load, so considerable amounts of bicarbonate are lost in the urine, and the serum bicarbonate level falls, resulting in a metabolic acidosis. The urine can still be acidified because distal hydrogen ion secretion is normal. Thus the acidic urinary pH is the clue that this is *proximal* renal tubular acidosis. Patients may present with faltering growth or vomiting.

5. C. Distal renal tubular acidosis

Distal (type 1) renal tubular acidosis is caused when the distal nephron cannot secrete hydrogen ions, thus preventing the reabsorption of the final 15% of bicarbonate. This causes a metabolic acidosis. However, the urinary pH cannot be reduced below about 5.5–6.0, even in the presence of severe systemic acidosis. If there is systemic metabolic acidosis, the body would usually try to compensate by producing acidic urine. In this case the urine cannot be acidified, which provides the clue to the diagnosis of *distal* renal tubular acidosis. Patients may present with urinary stones or nephrocalcinosis.

4) I, L, B, H, C

1. I. Exploratory surgery

This boy may have testicular torsion, which is an emergency, as any delay in providing appropriate treatment may cause infertility. An ultrasound scan should not be arranged, as this delays treatment. The child should undergo exploratory surgery with fixation of the testicles.

2. L. None of the above

This is most probably a hydrocoele, which is a collection of fluid around the testicle. It is fairly common in newborns, and the parents should be reassured that it will usually settle without treatment. It is important to ensure that the swelling is not a hernia, as this would require surgical management. A hydrocoele can be transilluminated, and the swelling is limited to the scrotal sac. In contrast, a hernia does not usually transilluminate, and will extend up to the inguinal canal.

3. B. Circumcision

This boy has phimosis (tightening of the foreskin), which is causing urinary obstruction. He needs an urgent urology opinion and most probably requires an urgent circumcision. If surgery has to be delayed for any reason, it may be necessary to place a catheter to relieve the urinary obstruction, but this is likely to be difficult to place due to the phimosis.

4. H. Upper pole hemi-nephrectomy

This girl has an ectopic ureter. In this condition the ureter attaches to an abnormal place, such as the urethra or vagina, instead of the bladder. In children with a duplex kidney the ectopic ureter is usually from the upper pole of the kidney, whereas the ureter from the lower pole usually drains correctly into the bladder. The key sign in the history is the child with constant dribbling day and night. There are several surgical options, one of which involves removing the upper pole of the kidney.

5. C. Advise against circumcision

This newborn has hypospadias. This condition occurs when the urethral opening is ectopically located on the ventral (lower) surface of the penis, proximal to the glans penis. It may even be located as far down as the scrotum or perineum. The penis is more likely to have associated ventral shortening and curvature (known as cordee) with more proximal urethral defects. Management involves surgical repair, which is required for cosmetic and functional reasons. The foreskin is used during the repair, so the parents must be advised not to get the child circumcised.

9 Emergency paediatrics and non-accidental injury

QUESTIONS

1) From the list of options below, please select the most appropriate initial management for each of the following scenarios concerning the management of paediatric emergencies. Each option may be used more than once.

   A. IV ceftriaxone
   B. Refer to plastic surgeon
   C. Intravenous saline bolus 30 ml/kg
   D. Abdominal thrusts
   E. Intubation
   F. Intravenous adrenaline
   G. Intraosseous needle in the distal tibia
   H. CT of the head
   I. Intraosseous needle in the proximal tibia
   J. FAST scan
   K. Back blows
   L. IM benzylpenicillin

   1. An 11-year-old boy presents with extensive burns caused by a house fire. He is alert but is crying and has a hoarse voice. Some of the burns are full thickness.

   2. A 2-year-old girl is unresponsive after being involved in a road traffic accident. Her main injury is bruising to her abdomen, and

her capillary refill time is 6 seconds. Attempts to place an intravenous cannula have been unsuccessful.

3. A 5-year-old boy presents to the Accident and Emergency department with a fever and a spreading non-blanching rash.

4. A 1-year-old boy was in the Accident and Emergency department waiting to be seen for a cut on his head when he started to choke on a crisp. He initially tried to cough, and he developed marked recession. However, his coughs became weaker and he has now become cyanosed.

5. A 5-year-old boy has multiple injuries after falling out of a second-floor window on to a wall. He has been intubated. His blood pressure is 70/30 mmHg and his pulse is 150 beats/minute.

2) From the list of options below, please select the most appropriate initial management for each of the following scenarios concerning acute allergic reactions and their differential diagnoses. Each option may be used more than once.

A. Intravenous antibiotics
B. Intravenous adrenaline
C. Chlorphenamine
D. Prednisolone
E. IM adrenaline
F. Intravenous hydrocortisone
G. Breathing into a paper bag
H. Intravenous salbutamol
I. Nebulised adrenaline
J. Dexamethasone
K. Oral antibiotics
L. Chloramphenicol eye drops

1. A 3-year-old girl suddenly develops stridor and a barking cough 90 minutes after eating her dinner. She is now struggling to breathe, with marked recession. Her oxygen saturations are 85% in air.

2. A 2-year-old girl develops tender erythematous swelling around her left eyelid. She has also had a fever, for which her mother has been giving her ibuprofen.

3. A 5-year-old boy develops swelling of his lips and tongue and an urticarial rash on his fingers shortly after eating some cake at a friend's birthday party. He is otherwise well.

4. A 7-year-old girl with a history of asthma that is difficult to control develops a widespread urticarial rash, severe wheeze and swelling of her lips and tongue shortly after eating a peanut.

5. An 11-year-old girl develops tachypnoea during lunchtime at school. Her blood gas analysis shows pH 7.47, CO_2 3.0 kPa and HCO_3^- 25 mmol/l. Her ammonia level is 25 micromol/l.

3) From the list of options below, please select the most likely diagnosis for each of the following scenarios concerning metabolic and endocrine emergencies. Each option may be used more than once.

A. Hyperglycaemia
B. Diabetic ketosis
C. Diabetes insipidus
D. Multiple endocrine neoplasia
E. Diabetic ketoacidosis
F. Fat oxidation disorder
G. Cerebral oedema
H. Congenital adrenal hypoplasia
I. Addisonian crisis
J. Diabetes mellitus
K. Sodium toxicity
L. Congenital adrenal hyperplasia

1. A 13-month-old girl presents with a tonic–clonic seizure lasting for 10 minutes. Her parents inform you that she has had diarrhoea and vomiting for 24 hours and is refusing meals. Her blood glucose level was found to be 0.5 mmol/l.

2. A 3-day-old boy presents very unwell with a capillary refill time of 6 seconds. He appears very quiet and is dehydrated. He was born by a normal delivery after prolonged rupture of membranes, and his newborn check was normal apart from the fact that he had hypospadias and bilaterally undescended testes.

3. A 15-year-old girl presented with diabetic ketoacidosis and was assessed to be 15% dehydrated. She received 30 ml/kg 0.9% sodium chloride bolus and was prescribed 0.9% sodium chloride at a rate that was calculated in order to rehydrate her over 24 hours. However, 6 hours into her treatment she complains of a headache and then becomes drowsy and confused.

4. A 14-year-old girl presents after a fainting episode. She has a blood pressure of 80/50mmHg, and appears to be 10–15% dehydrated. Her blood gas analysis shows pH 7.25, CO_2 4.0 kPa and HCO_3^- 18 mmol/l. Her sodium level is 125 mmol/l.

5. A 7-year-old boy presents with dehydration and breathlessness. His venous blood gas analysis shows pH 7.1, CO_2 3.5 kPa, HCO_3^- 15 mmol/l and base excess −10 mmol/l.

4) From the list of options below, please select the most appropriate initial action for each of the following scenarios concerning child protection issues. Each option may be used more than once.

   A. Ask the child if mummy hurt them
   B. Discharge with no follow-up
   C. Discharge with follow-up
   D. Phone the Children's Social Care Team
   E. Perform a coagulation screen
   F. Perform a blood test for full blood count
   G. Take photographs for evidence
   H. CT of the head
   I. Skull X-ray
   J. Ophthalmology review
   K. Skeletal survey
   L. Tell the parents that their child will probably be taken into care

1. A 5-year-old girl presents with a spiral humeral fracture. Her mother says that she tripped over the back step, but the girl looks nervous and says 'No I didn't, it was on purpose.'

2. A 3-month-old girl is brought to the Accident and Emergency department by her parents after having a fit at home. She is unconscious on arrival and then has a prolonged apnoea that requires intubation. Closer examination reveals that she has several small round bruises on her back and on her chest which are each about 1 cm in diameter.

3. A 4-month-old girl presents with a swelling on her left leg. She is otherwise well and alert. An X-ray reveals a spiral fracture of her left femur. Her parents tell you that they don't know how it occurred and that maybe her 18-month-old brother hit her. She has been seen by the orthopaedic team and is in traction, and they have already referred her to the Children's Social Care Team and to ophthalmology.

4. A 3-year-old girl who is in foster care due to neglect attends the Accident and Emergency department after the social worker noticed bruises on her at a routine visit. The foster mother says that she doesn't know how the girl got the bruises, and that she

must have been hit by another child in the household. The girl has not been to nursery recently as she has been unwell and complaining that her leg hurts. On examination, she looks pale and there is marked bruising on her left thigh, on both shins and on her right shoulder. She also has some petechial marks on her left shoulder and on her face.

5. A 2-year-old boy presents to the Accident and Emergency department with a mild viral upper respiratory tract infection. The triage nurse informs you that she is concerned because she noticed that he had a bruise on his forehead. You examine the boy and find a 2 cm yellow bruise on his forehead and three small bruises on his shin and knees. They are all different colours. His mother says that he hit his head on the corner of the dining table a few days ago and that he is very active and always bumping into things.

ANSWERS

1) E, I, A, K, J

1. E. Intubation

When managing extensive burns, the initial priority (as always) should be to focus on stabilisation of airway, breathing and circulation. Initial assessment is directed towards identifying any features that suggest airway involvement. These include singed nasal hairs or eyebrow hairs, carbonaceous sputum, barking cough, altered voice or respiratory distress. If stridor or hoarse voice is present, this indicates upper airway involvement, and early intubation is required before evolving oedema causes total obstruction. Delayed intubation in this setting is especially hazardous. Given that this child had third-degree burns, he will probably require a referral to a plastic surgeon, but this is not an immediate priority.

2. I. Intraosseous needle in the proximal tibia

Peripheral venous cannulation is often difficult when children are shocked and peripherally shut down. If fluid resuscitation or medication is needed immediately and venous cannulation is difficult, quick access can be obtained by placing an intraosseous needle into the antero-medial surface of the tibia, 2–3 cm below the tibial tuberosity. However, avoid limbs with fractures proximal to the insertion site.

3. A. IV ceftriaxone

Meningococcal sepsis should be suspected in any child with a fever and a spreading non-blanching rash. The appropriate initial in-hospital action would be to administer IV ceftriaxone. However, if you were a GP in the community, where you are unlikely to have ceftriaxone or any way of securing intravenous access, it would be appropriate to give intramuscular benzylpenicillin before sending the child immediately to the emergency department.

4. K. Back blows

This is perhaps a slightly unfair question for undergraduate examinations, as most medical schools provide only a few sessions on paediatric life support. However, foreign body airway obstruction is a common and important presentation, and every doctor should know how to manage it. A combination of back blows, chest thrusts and abdominal thrusts is utilised to relieve the obstruction. However, due to the lack of protection of the upper abdominal organs by the ribcage in smaller children, there is a risk of damage to these vital structures associated with the abdominal thrusts in particular. Therefore, especially in infants, it is best to use back blows and chest thrusts only. Note that chest thrusts are different to chest compressions, and take place at a slower rate, of about 1 thrust per second.

5. J. FAST scan

FAST (Focused Assessment by ultraSonography for Trauma) has been promoted as a quick and effective preliminary screening tool for evaluation of the abdomen in the traumatised child. Its aim is to detect free fluid/bleeding in the peritoneal cavity. The detection of free fluid in the child with deteriorating vital signs supports the decision to proceed with operative treatment. This child had a low blood pressure and was tachycardic, which suggests that he was developing shock, and the most likely cause of this was hypovolaemia secondary to intra-abdominal bleeding. If a FAST scan is not immediately available, an urgent CT of the abdomen would be appropriate. This child may well require some fluid resuscitation, but this would be by 10 ml/kg boluses with reassessment after each bolus. He probably also requires a CT of the head, but remember that cerebral oedema causes high blood pressure and bradycardia. If his blood pressure had been 130/90 mmHg and his heart rate had been 50 beats/minute, he would definitely have required an urgent CT of the head, and this would have been your priority.

2) I, A, C, E, G

1. I. Nebulised adrenaline

Stridor is a sign of upper respiratory tract obstruction (also known as upper airway obstruction), whereas wheeze is a sign of lower respiratory tract obstruction. A history of stridor and a barking cough in a child between 6 months and 6 years of age is most likely to be due to viral croup. Symptoms are usually worse in the late evening and at night. The virus causes oedema of the subglottic area, which results in narrowing of the upper airway, and consequently the child develops stridor and a barking cough. Most cases of moderate or severe croup can be treated with oral dexamethasone or nebulised steroids (budesonide), which reduce the severity and duration of the illness. However, this child clearly has very severe upper airway obstruction, and nebulised adrenaline can provide a transient immediate improvement in obstruction. This child should also receive oral dexamethasone, but the most appropriate initial action is to give an adrenaline nebuliser, as this will have a more immediate effect. In situations where nebulised adrenaline is required, intubation should be considered. Nebulised adrenaline has only a transient effect, and close monitoring is essential. It is unlikely that this child has had an anaphylactic reaction to her dinner, as it was consumed 90 minutes before any symptoms appeared, and she did not have any urticarial rash or swelling around her mouth.

2. A. Intravenous antibiotics

This child has periorbital cellulitis. This is unlikely to be an allergic reaction, as the erythema is tender and unilateral, and the child has a fever. The appropriate treatment for periorbital cellulitis is IV antibiotics, as if this condition is treated inadequately it can lead to orbital cellulitis, which can go on to cause meningitis or cavernous sinus thrombosis.

3. C. Chlorphenamine

This is typical of a local allergic reaction. Activation of mast cells causes the release of mediators, including histamine. This in turn leads to a local increase in the permeability of capillaries and venules, producing an urticarial rash. The swelling and rash have occurred at the sites that were in contact with the allergen (i.e. the hands and the mouth). Just because there is swelling in the mouth this does not mean that the reaction is a systemic one. If the allergen has come into contact with the mouth, this could be a local reaction. However, it is always important to check for other signs, such as hypotension or wheeze, which would point towards the reaction being an anaphylactic one. Local or mild allergic reactions can be treated with chlorphenamine (an antihistamine) and oral prednisolone. Chlorphenamine has a quicker onset of action, but doses may need to be repeated regularly. Prednisolone is a steroid and takes longer to exert an effect, so although it may be used in addition to chlorphenamine, the latter will probably produce a quicker result.

4. E. Intramuscular adrenaline

After removing the allergen, the most important treatment for moderate or severe allergic reactions is intramuscular adrenaline. IM adrenaline has a rapid onset of action, with peak levels being reached by 8 minutes. Other treatments can be given, depending on the signs present. If the child has wheeze, as in this case, they should also be given high-flow oxygen and nebulised salbutamol. If stridor is present, nebulised adrenaline can also be given. For hypotension, 20 ml/kg saline bolus can be given. Treatment of moderate or severe allergic reactions should also include antihistamines and steroids, but IM adrenaline and the treatments mentioned above are the most appropriate initial treatments. Steroids have a longer-lasting effect than adrenaline and chlorphenamine, and so help to prevent biphasic reactions. Biphasic reactions are defined as worsening of symptoms, that requires new therapy, after the resolution of anaphylaxis, and they occur in approximately 5% of children with anaphylaxis. The biphasic reaction usually occurs between 4 and 10 hours after the initial event. In this case the child had a background history of asthma. Allergies are more common in children with a history of asthma, and asthma sufferers tend to experience more severe bronchospasm when they have an allergic reaction.

5. G. Breathing into a paper bag

This blood gas analysis shows a respiratory alkalosis, i.e. a low CO_2 level is causing an alkaline pH value. If this continues, the low CO_2 level causes cerebral vasoconstriction. The most common cause of respiratory alkalosis is iatrogenic, due to overventilation of ventilated patients. However, given that this child is not being mechanically ventilated, the next most likely cause is hyperventilation due to anxiety. If the child breathes into a paper bag, the CO_2 level should increase to normal, as the exhaled air will have a higher CO_2 content. This does not alleviate the anxiety itself, but merely helps to correct the respiratory acidosis, and the cause of the anxiety will still need to be addressed. Respiratory alkalosis can also be caused by hyperammonaemia, as ammonia acts directly on the brainstem as a respiratory stimulant. Hyperammonaemia could be caused by a metabolic disorder such as a urea cycle defect. However, this child's ammonia level is normal (normal range is < 40 micromol/l).

3) F, L, G, I, E

1. F. Fat oxidation defect

A child with a fat oxidation disorder (e.g. medium-chain acyl-CoA dehydrogenase (MCAD) deficiency) needs to eat regularly to maintain their blood sugar levels. If a child with such a disorder has an episode of fasting or a vomiting illness, their sugar levels can become very low, and this may present as a hypoglycaemic seizure. It is therefore likely that this child had a fit due to hypoglycaemia which was caused by a fat oxidation disorder. Hypoglycaemia is defined as a blood sugar level of less than 2.6 mmol/l. Bedside glucose monitoring should be performed in all children who are unwell, as they are more prone to hypoglycaemia due to metabolic stress than adults.

2. L. Congenital adrenal hyperplasia

Congenital adrenal hyperplasia (CAH) is the most common non-iatrogenic cause of insufficient adrenal activity. The adrenal gland is responsible for producing cortisol, mineralocorticoids and sex hormones. There are many enzymes involved in the metabolic pathways that produce these three types of hormones. In CAH, one or more of the enzymes is deficient. Depending on which enzyme(s) are deficient, there will be a deficiency of the hormones produced by the enzyme(s), and a backlog (and therefore an increase) in substances that are normally used by the enzyme(s). The enzyme that is most commonly deficient is 21-hydroxylase, which is needed both in the pathway that produces mineralocorticoids and in the pathway that produces cortisol. Therefore a baby with 21-hydroxylase deficiency may present with a salt-losing crisis and a low blood pressure. There is also accumulation of the substances that would normally be acted on by the 21-hydroxylase, as their pathways are blocked. These excess substances spill over into the sex hormone pathway and cause excess amounts of testosterone to be produced. This is why some babies (especially girls) develop ambiguous genitalia. The baby in this scenario did not have any palpable testes and was diagnosed with hypospadias. It is likely that this baby is in fact a virilised girl with ambiguous genitalia, who then later presented with a salt-losing crisis and circulatory collapse. It is therefore very important that all babies with bilaterally unpalpable testes have their chromosomes checked. There was also a history of prolonged rupture of membranes prior to delivery, so sepsis must also be considered and treated while awaiting the results.

3. G. Cerebral oedema

The main danger associated with giving fluid replacement too quickly in diabetic ketoacidosis is cerebral oedema (due to decreasing intravascular osmolarity), which has developed in this patient. It occurs in 0.5% of children as a complication of diabetic ketoacidosis, and presents with a combination of neurological symptoms, including changes in conscious level, irritability, headache, cranial nerve palsies and seizures. Treatment is with IV mannitol and intubation. When rehydrating patients with diabetic ketoacidosis, it is best to give smaller boluses if required, usually 10 ml/ kg, and to correct the overall fluid deficit over a period of 48 hours, rather than 24 hours.

4. I. Addisonian crisis

This girl has a low blood pressure and is dehydrated. She has a partially compensated metabolic acidosis (pH is low and bicarbonate levels are low, therefore metabolic acidosis; CO_2 low, therefore partially compensated). However, the main clue to the cause of all this is that her sodium level is very low (normal range is 135–145 mmol/l). It is therefore most likely that she is having an addisonian crisis. This causes salt losing, hypoglycaemia, hypotension and eventually shock. Addison's disease is very rare in children, but it can be caused by an autoimmune process, sometimes associated with other autoimmune disorders.

5. E. Diabetic ketoacidosis

This boy has a severe partially compensated metabolic acidosis. He is breathless because by hyperventilating he can reduce his CO_2 level and therefore try to compensate for his metabolic acidosis. The most common cause of this presentation is diabetic ketoacidosis. He should have a bedside blood glucose test and blood ketones checked immediately. This will confirm the diagnosis.

4) D, H, K, F, B

1. D. Phone the Children's Social Care Team

In this case the best option on the list is to telephone the Children's Social Care Team to discuss your concerns. If you are a junior doctor in the hospital, you will have a Paediatric Registrar or Consultant whom you can contact, and they will often come to assess the child. However, if that option is not available, you can phone the Children's Social Care Team yourself and explain that you have concerns about child protection. It is best not to ask the child leading questions, such as 'Did mummy hurt you?' However, it is appropriate to ask very open questions, such as 'How did you get hurt?' or 'Can you tell me more about it?' Spiral fractures are often caused by twisting forces, and although they are seen more often in abuse, they are not diagnostic of the latter.

2. H. CT of the head

It is likely that this baby has been shaken, and a CT of the head is needed urgently in case any operative or medical treatment is required. The history of the fit and unconsciousness point to intracranial pathology, and the round bruises sound like fingertip bruises caused by squeezing the chest of the baby. Typically, fingertip bruises are small round bruises, with two on the front of the chest (from the adult thumbs) and eight on the back of the chest (from the fingers). However, variations are often seen. The baby should also have an ophthalmology review to look for retinal haemorrhages, and a skeletal survey to look for other injuries, but these are for diagnostic reasons, and will not affect the short-term management of this sick infant. Police and the Children's Social Care Team should also be contacted, but again this is not as urgent as a CT of the head.

3. K. Skeletal survey

A non-mobile child should not have bruises and certainly should not develop fractures unless there is a clear history of how they occurred. The story of the 18-month-old brother hitting this infant would not be consistent with a spiral fracture, which is caused by a twisting action, and a high level of force would need to have been used to cause such a fracture. This infant will require a skeletal survey, in which every bone in the body is X-rayed to check for other fresh or old fractures. It is important that this is done as soon as possible after admission, partly so that the parents cannot blame the staff for any other fractures that are found. A referral to the Children's Social Care Team and to ophthalmology to look for retinal haemorrhages (a sign that the child may have been shaken) is also appropriate, and this has already been done in this scenario.

4. F. Perform a blood test for full blood count

This child has multiple bruises and petechiae with no history or explanation. Of course non-accidental injury is possible, but in this case it is very important to rule out other causes of bruising, such as leukaemia or other bleeding disorders. This child has been feeling unwell for some time, and has complained of leg pain. It is therefore very important to rule out leukaemia by performing a full blood count and blood film. The patient's coagulation status should also be checked, but leukaemia is more likely with this history.

5. B. Discharge with no follow-up

Toddlers are often unstable on their feet, and it is usual for them to have a few bruises. The most common places are on bony prominences, such as the knees, shins, forehead and elbows. If the bruises are minor, the parents are acting appropriately and you are satisfied that the explanation given could have caused the injury, no further action is needed. However, red flags for non-accidental injuries are stories that change, delay in presentation, explanations that do not match the injuries, and injuries in non-mobile children. Also ask yourself whether the supervision of the child was appropriate at the time of the injury. Injuries in unusual places, such as the ear, mouth, back, chest, abdomen or inner aspects of the arms or legs should raise suspicion. If you are not sure, it is always better to discuss the case with your senior colleague.

10 Public health and statistics

QUESTIONS

1) From the list of options below, please select the most likely condition for each of the following statements concerning childhood mortality. Each option may be used more than once.

A. Childhood cancer
B. Injury and poisoning
C. Prematurity
D. Malaria
E. Sudden unexpected death in infancy
F. Pneumonia
G. Cerebral palsy
H. Congenital abnormalities
I. Arrhythmias and sudden cardiac arrest
J. Renal disease
K. Epilepsy
L. Diarrhoea

1. This is the leading cause of post-neonatal deaths in England and Wales.

2. This is the leading cause of death in children aged between 5 and 10 years in England and Wales.

3. This is the commonest cause of death in boys aged over 15 years.

4. This is the leading cause of death in children aged under 5 years worldwide.

5. This is the second commonest cause of death in children aged under 5 years worldwide.

2) From the list of options below, please select the most likely diagnosis for each of the following scenarios and statements concerning child-hood screening. Each option may be used more than once.

A. Down's syndrome
B. Congenital hypothyroidism
C. Phenylketonuria
D. Cystic fibrosis
E. Sickle-cell disease
F. Duchenne muscular dystrophy
G. Congenital cataract
H. Hearing impairment
I. Juvenile idiopathic arthritis
J. Edwards' syndrome
K. MCADD
L. Cervical cancer

1. At her booking visit a 42-year-old pregnant mother asks you about antenatal screening. You discuss with her a particular condition for which a prenatal screening test is routinely offered nationally.

2. A pregnant mother has recently met a severely disabled teen-ager with this genetic condition, and is very concerned that her unborn child might have it. She wants to know whether it can be routinely screened for. You explain that it is not part of the national screening programme.

3. A 2-week-old boy has been diagnosed with this condition fol-lowing the neonatal blood spot test. His parents are being counselled about a strict diet, which he must adhere to.

4. This condition is screened for as part of the neonatal check per-formed by the paediatrician on each baby during the first few days of life. It requires a specialised piece of equipment.

5. This condition has an autosomal recessive inheritance pattern and is screened for on the neonatal blood spot test (heel prick test), which if positive would show high levels of immunoreac-tive trypsinogen.

3) From the list of options below, please select the most likely condition for each of the following scenarios concerning notifiable diseases. Each option may be used more than once.

A. Tuberculosis
B. Meningitis
C. Mumps
D. Food poisoning
E. Chickenpox
F. Measles
G. Rubella
H. Viral hepatitis
I. Malaria
J. Whooping cough
K. Cholera
L. Anthrax

1. Five children in the same nursery class contract the same disease. The GP says that it is not a notifiable condition.

2. A 17-year-old boy contracts this illness. He sees his GP as he has read on the Internet that it could render him infertile, and he is very concerned about this.

3. A 26-year-old pregnant woman contracts this condition during pregnancy. Her baby is born with growth retardation, visual problems, hearing impairment and a patent ductus arteriosus.

4. A 10-year-old boy presents to the Accident and Emergency department feeling generally unwell. He is complaining of a headache, myalgia and an intermittent fever over the last few days. He has recently returned from visiting relatives in India.

5. A GP sees a 5-year-old girl who has been coryzal and feverish. She has Koplik spots in her mouth. A few days later she develops a macular rash all over her trunk.

4) From the list of options below, please select the term being described by each of the following statements concerning commonly used statistical terminology. Each answer may be used more than once.

A. Incidence
B. Rate
C. Specificity
D. Prevalence
E. Absolute risk reduction
F. Risk ratio
G. Sensitivity
H. Number needed to treat
I. Positive predictive value
J. Odds ratio
K. Negative predictive value
L. Numerator

1. This term describes the number of children who develop Henoch–Schönlein purpura per year in the UK.

2. This term describes the number of children living with cystic fibrosis in the UK in January 2010.

3. This term describes the proportion of newborn babies with congenital hypothyroidism who are correctly identified by the neonatal blood spot test.

4. This term describes the proportion of babies without cystic fibrosis who have a negative neonatal immunoreactive trypsinogen test.

5. This term describes the effectiveness of a therapeutic healthcare intervention. Its value is equal to the inverse of the absolute risk reduction.

ANSWERS

1) H, A, B, F, L

1. H. Congenital abnormalities

The term 'post-neonatal death' refers to a death that occurs between 28 days and 1 year of life. The most common cause in this category is congenital abnormalities, for which the spectrum of severity is vast. This is partly due to the array of systems that can be affected, but also depends on the nature of the defects themselves. In some cases, children may have multiple congenital abnormalities, and their life expectancy is shortened as a result.

2. A. Childhood cancer

Childhood cancer is the leading cause of death in children aged between 5 and 10 years. Despite this, about 75% of childhood cancer patients in the UK currently survive for at least 5 years after diagnosis. Patients with retinoblastoma, gonadal germ-cell tumours and Hodgkin's lymphoma do particularly well, with 5-year survival rates of about 95%. Only one of the common diagnostic groups, primitive neuroectodermal tumours, had a recent 5-year survival rate of less than 50%.

3. B. Injury and poisoning

As children get older they have increasing scope to make their own decisions. They start to partake in more risk-prone activities, such as experimenting with tobacco, alcohol and illicit drugs, joyriding and performing extreme sports. These changes are reflected in the injuries and problems with which they present.

4. F. Pneumonia

Pneumonia is the commonest cause of mortality in children under 5 years old on a worldwide basis, and accounts for 19% of these deaths. It is particularly common and often life-threatening in the developing world. Many of these children have not received any vaccinations, so are at higher risk of contracting infections in the first place. In addition to this, it is obviously more difficult to obtain access to healthcare, oxygen, adequate hydration and antibiotics, and as a result many of these infants succumb to this illness.

5. L. Diarrhoea

Diarrhoea is the second commonest cause of mortality in children under 5 years old on a worldwide basis. It is an incredibly common problem in the developing world. Inexpensive and effective treatments for diarrhoea exist, such as oral rehydration therapy or intravenous fluids, but in developing countries children often have no access to such treatment.

2) A, F, C, G, D

1. A. Down's syndrome

The national antenatal Down's syndrome screening programme aims to ensure that all pregnant women are offered the tests and can make informed choices about pregnancy outcome. This is to reduce the number of babies who are born with undiagnosed Down's syndrome. A number of tests exist, and others are being developed. These include maternal serum markers such as AFP, beta-hCG, inhibin-A and unconjugated oestradiol, as well as ultrasound scanning for nuchal translucency. These tests enable clinicians to establish the risk of Down's syndrome. If this risk exceeds 1 in 250, women are offered further cytogenetic tests, such as amniocentesis or chorionic villus sampling. Based on this information they can make an informed choice about how to proceed.

2. F. Duchenne muscular dystrophy

This is an X-linked recessive disorder which affects 1 in 4000 males. It generally presents in early childhood and progresses throughout childhood. Life expectancy is shortened considerably, with affected males generally only surviving into their teens to early twenties. In 2004 the National Screening Committee assessed the condition against its criteria, and it was not recommended that a national screening programme be adopted. However, affected families can be offered prenatal genetic testing.

3. C. Phenylketonuria

Phenylketonuria is an autosomal recessive condition, and was the first disease to become part of the newborn screening programme. The incidence is 1 in 100 000. It is characterised by a deficiency of the hepatic enzyme phenylalanine hydroxylase, which is necessary to metabolise the amino acid phenylalanine. The accumulation of this amino acid leads to progressive irreversible neurological damage. Starting a strict low-phenylalanine diet during the first 2–3 weeks of life can prevent these devastating symptoms.

4. G. Congenital cataract

All neonates undergo a full clinical examination that acts as a screening tool for a number of congenital abnormalities. Congenital cataracts are screened for using an ophthalmoscope. The absence of the red reflex should alert the examiner to a possible diagnosis. Other congenital disorders that are screened for at the newborn check include congenital heart disease, developmental dislocation of the hips and other congenital malformations.

5. D. Cystic fibrosis

Cystic fibrosis is an autosomal recessive condition, and 1 in 25 people carry a mutated version of the gene. Biochemical screening for cystic fibrosis uses a technique that identifies raised levels of immunoreactive trypsinogen (IRT) and allows early detection and diagnosis of the condition. If the test shows high levels of IRT, the diagnosis is confirmed with a sweat test or with genetic testing.

3) E, C, G, I, F

1. E. Chickenpox

Chickenpox is a common childhood infection caused by the spread of varicella zoster virus. It is contagious from 48 hours before the spots occur until all of the spots have crusted over. Complications can include superimposed bacterial infection, pneumonia, neonatal varicella and encephalitis. Immunocompromised children should receive zoster immunoglobulin as soon as possible (within 96 hours) after contact.

2. C. Mumps

Since the much publicised concerns about the MMR vaccine, the incidence of mumps has started to increase. Mumps is generally a self-limiting illness which causes pain and swelling of the parotid glands, but in males it can cause orchitis, which in turn can lead to infertility in some cases.

3. G. Rubella

Rubella is a viral infection, which can be sub-clinical. If symptoms do occur, patients complain of lymphadenopathy, mild fever and coryza, arthralgia and a rash. Contracting rubella in the early stages of pregnancy can be highly teratogenic, causing intrauterine growth restriction, congenital heart defects, sensorineural hearing loss, congenital cataracts, mental retardation and other significant problems.

4. I. Malaria

Malaria is a disease that is spread by the female *Anopheles* mosquito. The condition is not endemic in the UK, but cases are seen in travellers returning to this country. Symptoms include fever and rigors (which are typically cyclical), arthralgia, headache, vomiting, anaemia and convulsions. A blood film showing malaria parasites confirms the diagnosis. Prevention of this condition is essential, and travellers must be counselled about the risks and advised about the use of mosquito nets, repellent and malaria prophylaxis.

5. F. Measles

Measles generally starts with a coryzal illness, fever and conjunctivitis. Koplik spots are pathognomonic of the condition, and develop inside the mouth a day or so later, but are not always seen. A macular rash usually develops afterwards, starting on the head and neck and slowly spreading across the body. It is usually self-limiting and lasts about 7–10 days. Measles encephalitis is the most serious and potentially devastating complication, as it can lead to serious brain damage.

4) A, D, G, C, H

1. A. Incidence

Incidence refers to the number of new cases in a particular population over a particular time frame. It is often represented as a proportion. For example, the estimated annual incidence of Henoch–Schönlein purpura in the UK is 20 in 100 000.

2. D. Prevalence

Prevalence refers to the total number of individuals with a particular disease at a particular point in time. For example, the prevalence of cystic fibrosis in the UK is 1 in 2500.

3. G. Sensitivity

When designing a test it is important to keep the number of false negatives and false positives as low as possible. Sensitivity is a measure of how well a test can accurately detect people who are truly affected by the disease. It is calculated by dividing the number of affected people with a positive test result (true positives) by the total number of people with the disease (true positives and false negatives). A test with a low sensitivity produces a large number of false negatives (i.e. it misses a large number of cases).

4. C. Specificity

It is also important that a test can correctly identify people who are truly unaffected by the disease. Specificity is calculated by dividing the number of unaffected individuals with a negative test result (true negatives) by the total number of unaffected individuals (true negatives and false positives). A test with a low specificity produces a large number of false positives.

5. H. Number needed to treat

The number needed to treat (NNT) represents the number of people who need to be treated in order to prevent one adverse outcome. It is the inverse of the absolute risk reduction. The ideal NNT would be 1, where every individual has improved with the treatment. The higher the NNT, the less effective the treatment.

Index

21-hydroxylase   111

ABO blood group incompatibility   9
absent factor VIII   82
absolute risk reduction   125
acid-fast bacilli (AFB)   62
acquired immunodeficiency syndrome (AIDS)   33
ACTH (adrenocorticotropic hormone)   42
acute allergic reactions   101, 108–9
acute epiglottitis   35, 60
acute lymphoblastic leukaemia   83–4
acute post-streptococcal glomerulonephritis   93
Addisonian crisis   112
adrenaline   108, 109
AIDS (acquired immunodeficiency syndrome)   33
allergic reactions   35, 101, 108–9
ambiguous genitalia   85, 91, 111
amniocentesis   122
amphotericin   83
anaemia   80, 82
anal fissure   45
anaphylactic reaction   108, 109
Anopheles mosquito   29, 124
antenatal screening   117, 122
antihistamine   109
antistreptolysin O titre (ASOT)   93
aplastic anaemia   80
apnoeas   8, 59
appendicitis   44–5
arginine vasopressin (AVP)   93
arthritis   71
artificial ventilation   59
Asperger's syndrome   18
aspirin   44
asthma   61, 109
atrial septal defect (ASD)   58
autism   18

Bacillus cereus   48
back blows   106–7

bacterial endocarditis   58
bacterial peritonitis   34
barium enema   11
benign murmur   56
benzylpenicillin   106
beta thalassaemia major   82
bicarbonate   95
bilirubin   4, 9, 10
biochemical disturbances   88–9, 95–6
biphasic reactions   109
bisphosphonates   68
Blalock–Taussig (BT) shunt   59
blood group incompatibility   9
boot-shaped heart   52
Bordetella pertussis   60
Borrelia afzelii   71
bowed legs (genu varum)   70, 95
bowel movements   39, 44–5
bradycardia   2
bronchiolitis   60–1, 62
bruises   104–5, 113, 114
budesonide   108
burns   99, 106

Caesarean section   1, 4, 6
caffeine therapy   8
Campylobacter infections   48, 71
cancer   35, 120
candidiasis   26
cardiac disorders   51–2, 53, 56–9
cardiology and respiratory disease   51–62
   questions   51–5
   answers   56–62
causes of death   115–16
cavernous sinus thrombosis   108
ceftriaxone   106
central cyanosis   1
central diabetes insipidus   93
cerebral oedema   112
cerebral palsy   18, 35
cervical cancer   35
chemotherapy   77, 83, 84
chest thrusts   106–7

chickenpox 31, 124
childhood cancer 120
childhood gastroenteritis 41, 48–9
childhood malignancies 73–4, 78–9
childhood mortality 115–16, 120–1
childhood screening 117, 122–3
child protection issues 104–5, 113–14
Chlamydia trachomatis 71
chlorphenamine 109
choreoathetoid cerebral palsy 10
chorionic villus sampling 122
Christmas disease 77, 83
chromosomes 91, 111
chronic lung disease (CLD) 8
circumcision 97
cirrhosis 82
cleft palate 11
Clostridium botulinum 48
Clostridium difficile 71
coarctation of the aorta 56
coeliac disease 33, 47
complex partial seizures 22
congenital abnormalities 120
congenital adrenal hyperplasia (CAH) 111
congenital cataract 11, 122
congenital heart disease 123
constitutional growth delay (CGD) 42
cordee 97
cortisol 42
cow's milk intolerance 33
Craig splint 68
craniopharyngioma 20
crawling 21
croup (viral laryngotracheobronchitis) 29,
108
CT scan (computed tomography) 75, 82,
107, 113
cyanosis 1, 6, 53, 57, 100
cystic fibrosis 11, 46, 62, 119, 123, 125
cystic hygroma 5

dactylitis 72
deafness 18
delta F508 mutation 46
deprivation dwarfism 43
desmopressin 83
developmental dysplasia of the hip 68, 123
developmental milestones 16, 21
dexamethasone 108
diabetes 70, 82, 93
diabetic ketoacidosis 102, 112
diarrhoea 93, 121
Di George syndrome 95
diphtheria 35
distal (type 1) renal tubular acidosis 95–6
Down's syndrome 122
Duchenne muscular dystrophy 122
duct-dependent coarctation of the aorta 56

duplex kidney 90, 97

E. coli 34, 93
ectopic ureter 97
Edwards' syndrome 6–7
egg allergy 35
Eisenmenger's syndrome 56
ejection systolic murmur 51, 56
emergency paediatrics and non-accidental
injury 99–114
questions 99–105
answers 106–14
endocrine emergencies 102–3, 111–12
enuresis 90
epiglottitis 29, 35, 60
epilepsy 42
Epstein–Barr virus (EBV) 31, 80
Erb's palsy 11
erythema infectiosum 31
Escherichia coli 71
Ewing's sarcoma 78

faltering growth 37–8, 42–3, 52
FAST (Focused Assessment by
ultraSonography for Trauma) scan 107
fat oxidation disorder 111
febrile convulsions 19
femoral pulses 52
ferritin 82
fetal haemoglobin (HbF) 82
fetal hydrops 9
fifth disease 31
fingertip bruises 113
focal seizures 22
food poisioning 48
foreign body airway obstruction 61, 106–7
foreskin 90, 97
fractures 104, 113
Friedreich's ataxia 70
functional murmur 56

gastroenteritis 41, 48–9, 71
gastroenterology and endocrinology 37–49
questions 37–41
answers 42–9
gender 91
genetic testing 122, 123
genitalia 85, 90, 91, 92, 97, 111
genito-urinary problems in neonates 85–6,
91–2
genu valgum (knock-knees) 70, 88, 95
genu varum (bowed legs) 70, 95
Giardia lamblia 48
giardiasis 48
glandular fever 31
glucose-6-phosphate (G6PD) dehydrogenase
deficiency 9
gluten 47

gonadal germ-cell tumours   120
Group A streptococci   29, 71
Guillain–Barré syndrome   48

haematocrit   82
haematology and oncology   73–84
        questions   73–7
        answers   78–84
haemochromatosis   82
haemoglobin   80, 81, 82, 83
haemolysis   9
haemolytic uraemic syndrome   93
haemophilia   82, 83
Haemophilus influenzae   32, 35, 60
headache   15, 20
heart block   2, 7
heart murmurs   51, 52, 56
heel prick test   117
Henoch–Schönlein purpura   119, 125
hernia   97
Hib vaccine (*Haemophilus influenzae* type B)   35, 60
histamine   108
HIV (human immunodeficiency virus)   33
Hodgkin's lymphoma   120
homovanillic acid (HVA)   78
HPV (human papillomavirus)   35
human immunodeficiency virus (HIV)   33
hydrocoele   97
hydrops fetalis   9
hyperammonaemia   110
hyperbilirubinaemia   9
hypercapnoea   53, 59
hyperphosphataemia   95
hypertension   20
hyperventilation   109
hypocalcaemia   88–9, 95
hypoglycaemia   111
hypoparathyroidism   95
hypophosphataemia   95
hypospadias   97
hypotension   109

idiopathic thrombocytopenic purpura (ITP)   80
IgG antibodies   9
immune system disease   26–7, 33–4
immunisation   28, 35
immunoglobulin   34
immunology and infectious disease   23–35
questions   23–8
answers   29–35
immunoreactive trypsinogen (IRT)   117, 119, 123
incidence (definition)   125
infantile polycystic kidney disease   37, 42
infantile spasms   22

infectious disease *see* immunology and infectious disease
infectious mononucleosis (glandular fever)   31
infective bacterial endocarditis   58
infertility   97, 124
influenza   29
inhaled foreign body   61, 106–7
injuries   104–5, 113–14, 120
innocent murmur   56
intramuscular adrenaline   109
intubation   59, 106, 108
intussusception   44
iron   82
iron-deficiency anaemia   80
irritable hip   68

jaundice   4, 9
joint pain   66, 71
Jones criteria   71
juvenile idiopathic arthritis (JIA)   33
juvenile myoclonic epilepsy   22
juvenile psoriatic arthritis   72

Kawasaki disease   72
kernicterus   10
knock-knees (genu valgum)   70, 88, 95
Koplik spots   31, 118, 124
kwashiorkor   42–3

laryngomalacia   62
leukaemia   83–4, 114
limb problems   63–4, 68–9
lower urinary tract infection   93
Lyme disease   71

malaria   81, 124
malignancies   73–4, 78–9
Mantoux test   62
marasmus   42, 43
measles   31, 35, 124
measles encephalitis   124
Meckel's diverticulum   44
meconium   5, 11
medium-chain acyl-CoA dehydrogenase (MCAD) deficiency   111
meningitis   14, 18, 29, 31–2, 108
meningococcal sepsis   31, 106
menorrhagia   77
metabolic acidosis   95–6, 112
metabolic alkalosis   46
metabolic and endocrine emergencies   102–3, 111–12
methadone   6
micturating cysto-urethrogram (MCUG)   91
migraine   20
MMR (measles, mumps, rubella) vaccine   35, 124

moderate unilateral renal pelvis
  dilatation 85
Moro reflex 5, 11
mortality 115–16, 120–1
mumps 35, 124
murmurs 51, 52, 56
musculoskeletal deformities 65, 70
Mycobacterium tuberculosis 29
myocardial infarction 72
myoclonic jerks 22

naevus 17
naso-pharyngeal aspirate 62
National Screening Committee 122
nebulised adrenaline 108, 109
necrotising enterocolitis (NEC) 8
Neisseria meningitidis 31
neonatal abstinence syndrome (NAS) 6
neonatal blood spot test 117, 119
neonatal lupus erythematosus 7
neonatology 1–11
    questions 1–5
    answers 6–11
nephrology and urology 85–97
    questions 85–90
    answers 91–7
nephrotic syndrome 34, 94
neuroblastoma 78
neurofibromatosis 70
neurological problems in childhood 13–14,
  18–19
neurology and development 13–22
    questions 13–17
    answers 18–22
neutropenic sepsis 83
NNT *see* number needed to treat
non-accidental injuries 104–5, 113–14
non-paralytic strabismus 18
non-steroidal anti-inflammatory drugs 68
normocytic, normochromic anaemia 82
notifiable diseases 118, 124
number needed to treat (NNT) 125

oliguria 3
oncology *see* haematology and oncology
ophthalmoscopy 5
oral rehydration therapy 121
orbital cellulitis 108
orbital rhabdomyosarcoma 79
orthopaedics and rheumatology 63–72
    questions 63–7
    answers 68–72
Ortolani's test 63
Osgood–Schlatter disease 72
Osler's nodes 58
osteogenesis imperfecta 68–9
osteosarcoma 77, 78
otitis media 19

paediatric emergencies 99–100, 106–7
pansystolic murmur 52, 56
parainfluenza 29
partial seizures 22
patent ductus arteriosus (PDA) 8, 58
pathogens 23–4, 29–30
Pavlik harness 68
penis 90, 97
periorbital cellulitis 108
persistent pulmonary hypertension 57
Perthes' disease 68
pertussis 60
pes cavus (arched foot) 70
phenylalanine hydroxylase (PAH) 46, 122
phenylketonuria (PKU) 46, 122
phototherapy 4, 10
phymosis 97
physiological jaundice 9
physiological murmur 56
physiotherapy 68
pin fixation 68
PKU *see* phenylketonuria
Plasmodium falciparum 29
pneumococcal meningitis 18
pneumococcus 31
Pneumocystis carinii pneumonia 26, 33
pneumonia 26, 33, 120
poisoning 120
polio 35
polycythaemia 82
poor growth 40, 46–7
positional talipes 70
posterior urethral valve 91
post-neonatal death 115, 120
prednisolone 109
premature neonates 3, 8
prenatal screening 117
prevalence (definition) 125
primary hypoparathyroidism 95
primary polycythaemia 82
primitive neuroectodermal tumours 120
prostaglandin 1, 6, 53, 58, 59
protein-dominant malnutrition 42–3
proximal (type 2) renal tubular acidosis 95
psoriasis 72
public health and statistics 115–25
    questions 115–19
    answers 120–5
pulmonary hypertension 56, 57
pulse rate 53
pyelonephritis 93
pyloric stenosis 46

rash 25, 26, 101, 106, 108
reactive arthritis 71
red reflex 5, 11, 122
reflex anoxic seizure 22
Reiter's syndrome 71

renal failure 42
renal pelvis dilatation 85, 91
renal problems in neonates 85–6, 91–2
renal tubular acidosis 95–6
respiratory alkalosis 109–10
respiratory conditions 54, 55, 60–2
respiratory syncytial virus (RSV) 29, 60, 62
retinal haemorrhages 113–14
retinoblastoma 11, 78, 120
retinopathy of prematurity (ROP) 8
Reye's syndrome 44
rhabdomyosarcoma 78–9
Rhesus disease 9, 10
rheumatic fever 71
rheumatological problems 67, 72
rickets 70, 95
rocker-bottom foot 2, 6
rotavirus 49
RSV see respiratory syncytial virus
rubella 35, 124

salbutamol 109
scarlet fever 29–30
Scheuermann's disease 72
scoliosis 70
screening 117, 122–3
scrotal sac 90, 97
secondary lactase deficiency 46
secondary polycythaemia 82
seizures 17, 19, 22
sensitivity (definition) 125
sensorineural deafness 18
septic arthritis 29, 68, 71
severe bilateral renal pelvis dilatation 85
severe combined immunodeficiency (SCID) 33
sex hormones 111
Shiga toxin 93
short stature 37–8, 42–3
sickle-cell anaemia 80–1
sickle-cell crisis 83
simple partial seizures 22
skeletal survey 113
skin infections 25, 31–2
slapped cheek syndrome 31
slipped upper femoral epiphysis (SUFE) 68
sodium valproate 22
specificity (definition) 125
speech 21
spiral fractures 104, 113
splenectomy 80
splinter haemorrhages 53, 58
sputum microscopy 62
squint 13, 18
Staphylococcus aureus 29, 48, 71
statistical terminology 119, 125
steroids 84, 108, 109
stillbirth 2

Still's disease 72
strabismus (squint) 13, 18
Streptococcus 93
Streptococcus pneumoniae 34
stridor 60, 108, 109
Sturge–Weber disease 22
supraventricular tachycardia (SVT) 58
sweat test 11, 62, 123
systemic lupus erythematosus 7
systemic metabolic acidosis 96

tachypnoea 52
talipes equinovarus 70
TB see tuberculosis
temporo-mandibular dysfunction 20
tension headache 20
testicles 90, 92, 97
testicular torsion 97
testosterone 111
tetanus 35
tetralogy of Fallot 53, 56–7, 59
tonic–clonic seizures 19, 22, 102
transferrin 82
transient synovitis 68
transient tachypnoea of the newborn (TTN) 6
transposition of the great arteries (TGA) 6, 58
trisomy 18 6–7
tuberculosis (TB) 29, 62
tumour lysis syndrome 84
Turner's syndrome 11

undescended testicles 86, 92
upper pole hemi-nephrectomy 97
urinary tract infection 15, 86, 93
urine multistick 85–7, 93–4
urological problems 90, 97

vaccinations 120
vanillylmandelic acid (VMA) 78
varicella zoster virus (chickenpox) 31, 124
ventilation 59
ventricular septal defect (VSD) 56, 58, 82
verocytotoxin 93
vesico-ureteric reflux 91
viral croup 29, 108
vitamin D deficiency 70, 95
Von Willebrand's disease 83
VSD see ventricular septal defect

walking 21
West syndrome 38, 42
wheeze 60, 108, 109
whooping cough 60
Wilms' tumour 78
windswept knees 70
Wolf–Parkinson–White pre-excitation syndrome 58